Think And Grow Thin

By Thyra Samter Winslow

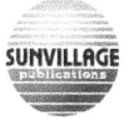

www.sunvillagepublications.com

Think And Grow Thin
By Thyra Samter Winslow

Copyright © 2010

No part of this publication may be reproduced, stored in a retrieval
system or transmitted in any form or by any means, electronic,
mechanical, photocopying, recording or otherwise, without prior written
permission from the publisher.

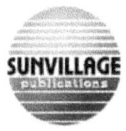

www.sunvillagepublications.com

Cover design by www.WebCopyAlchemy.com

Dedicated

to everyone connected with the manufacturing, distributing or publicizing of,

Avocadoes,
Bakery products,
Baked beans,
Butter,
Candy,
Cereals,
Cream,
Cheeses, the rich kinds,
Chocolate,
Dried fruit,
Fats,
Frozen fruit, with added sugar,
Ice cream,
Jellies and marmalades,
Liquors,
Margarine,
Oils,
Salt,
Sugar and
Wine.

I love you all, serve your products to my friends, recommend you to normal-weight people, and hope that this book will enable all overweights to think themselves thin enough to enjoy your delectable products.

CONTENTS

Foreword

BY DR. SIDNEY M. SCHNITTKE

THE MAJORITY OF PATIENTS who consult their physicians primarily because of obesity usually do so because they are confronted with a physical disfigurement. The dress that no longer hangs correctly and bulges in the wrong places, the pair of slacks that won't button around the waist comfortably; these are mute reminders that the body is acquiring excess poundage. The medical practitioner attacks the problem of primary obesity with great vigor—and usually with as great a lack of success.

This failure to secure results in reducing human obesity stems from two misconceptions. The patient considers his weight a cosmetic tragedy, and when he is told by his medical advisor that obesity is a disease fraught with perilous repercussions, he is wont to assume that the physician is trying to "scare him into reducing," and thus never considers the problem in its true light.

The physician errs when he approaches obesity simply as a disease process—an evidence of a disordered metabolism—and nothing more. Basically, it is such a pathological process, but it has superimposed overtones of addiction which take it out of the realm of ordinary illness. Just as a narcotic addict makes repeated vows to abandon his enslavement and attempts numerous "cures," so does the obese patient continually back-slide after self exhortations, and imposed injunctions have produced a temporary recession in the mounting weight indicator.

Let us consider another facet of this addiction; the patient who consults a doctor secondarily for obesity, i.e. a complaint wherein the overweight condition complicates a primary disorder such as hypertension, diabetes, etc., should certainly prove more amenable to the admonitions of the medical adviser. This patient has reached a terminal phase of the dire prognosis held out to the individual who consulted the physician simply for obesity—he or she now has visible evidence of the deleterious effects of the excess flesh. This state of affairs does not require foresight on the part of the patient to comprehend the eventual outcome of the disorder. He or she *must* lose weight in order to maintain life; yet a walk through any of the medical wards in a hospital will show the majority of patients afflicted with hypertension to be overweight. In this connection it is interesting that almost 65% of 200 practicing physicians over 40, examined for heart trouble, were obese, as revealed in a study released in May, 1951, by Dr. Arthur M. Master and Dr. Kenneth Chesky, both of New York City.

These individuals can see both by the scale reading and their comparative feeling of well-being that a loss of weight is accompanied by a corresponding decline in blood pressure. However, a goodly percentage of these addicts will go off their diet regimens repeatedly, re-elevate their blood pressure and commence again to suffer the tortures of the damned.

To my mind this book represents a great advance in the struggle against overweight. The author has set herself the task of acquainting the obese reader with the known facts concerning his malady; *why* he is overweight, *why* this excess poundage is dangerous, *why* it is really never too late to cast off the superfluous tissue, and lastly, how to achieve the desired reduction in a safe and sane fashion.

Since the therapy of obesity requires a reorientation of the mental outlook, it can readily be seen that the physician must enlist the patient's cooperation in order to achieve results. This book serves as an admirable adjunct to the office visit in that it expands upon and carries forward the idea that the patient *must* reduce. The physician who recommends this text to his patient is then assured of a continual flow of therapy much akin to that of a repository injection, and with the same effect.

This is not a spectacular book. In discussing obesity, Mrs. Winslow steers clear of the temptation to discourse concerning constipation, fatigue, faddist diets, etc. She means the text to apply only to the reader interested in losing weight. She makes one point quite clear; the obese person must watch his or her diet from now and forevermore. This is a simple truism and yet is as necessary as telling a reclaimed alcoholic that in the future he cannot imbibe with impunity from the cup that cheers.

In closing, I would remind the reader from my own experience of some ten thousand obese patients that there is only one cause for overweight—overeating I The causes for overeating are legion; and the identification of the reason why you continually cram more food than you need into your stomach is a prime requisite for the "cure" of obesity. The author of this work does not try to *cure* obesity—that the patient must do for himself— but she does offer a helping hand to the sincere seeker for aid in combating his problem.

CHAPTER I

It's later

than you think

WE WOULD ALL LIKE TO BE SLIM and young and good-looking. I wish I could wave a magic wand and transform all of you into glamorous, radiant creatures of twenty-one. But like the witch in John van Druten's *Bell, Book and Candle,* my wand is useless, and my broom, good only for prosaic, utilitarian tasks, stands idly in the closet. However, if you are overweight, I believe I can show you how to become comfortably thin, look and feel younger and healthier—and have a good chance to live longer, too, if you'll put your mind to it.

There are nearly one hundred and ten million adults in America, and it has been estimated that, of that number, over twenty-two million weigh too much—and would be better off if they didn't. When twenty per cent of a population suffers from a serious defect, something should be done about it. I'm not optimistic enough to believe that I can influence the weight and health of that great a portion of the population—but if I help even a few, I'll be mighty happy about it.

I'm taking it for granted that you weigh too much, or that someone you're interested in weighs too much.

1

Otherwise you'd be pretty foolish to waste your time over this book. Of course, you could gloat over the overweights and what they have to put up with! But this book is not for gloaters. It is for those who are too fat and who want to do something about it.

I could make definite promises that you'll lose weight—and look and feel better if you follow the rules you'll read here; I could guarantee that you'd weigh less and improve in health—but I don't dare. Not because you won't lose weight if you follow the rules, but because too many readers can't or won't read.

A few months ago, I wrote an article for the monthly magazine, *Your Life*. It contained rules for a simple self-analysis, based on the writing of a news story. I did not tell the readers to send me their analyses—but a lot of them must have thought I did, because they sent them in. And in practically every case they disregarded every rule I'd given, and seemingly forgot why they were writing or what they were writing about. And the other day a man I'd thought most intelligent said to me, "Weight reduction is all nonsense! I'm trying to reduce and I'm gaining, instead."

"What are you doing about it?" I asked.

"I'm following the Hauser rules and I've gained five pounds."

I asked for details.

"I just follow my regular meals," he said. "I haven't got time to diet. But each morning I have a glass of milk with blackstrap molasses mixed in it—and I tell you, I gained instead of lost weight."

Now, Gayelord Hauser's books are good. He's written three: *The Gayelord Hauser Cook Book, Diet Does It,* and *Look Younger, Live Longer.* I shall have more to say about them, and about other excellent books on diet. I believe that anyone who wants to lose weight should read a number of books about it—and get something out of each book. Of course, I think I've got something here that the others haven't got—or I wouldn't be writing this! Mr. Hauser recommends black molasses, but nowhere does he say that milk and black molasses, consumed in addition to a too-generous diet will take off weight. An eight-ounce glass of milk with several table-spoonfuls of black molasses will add about 250 calories to the daily intake—or almost a third of what is usually recommended in a strict diet for a whole day's rationing. So you see what I mean?

Of course, you aren't that kind of a reader! You understand what you read. And in order to get thin, you're going to follow, to the letter, exactly what I recommend. If you do, you'll find you'll lose weight easily and satisfactorily. Otherwise I don't want to hear from you, because it will mean you haven't followed the rules.

Why should you get thin ? You may know the answers as well as I do. Or you may not know all of them.

First of all, but far from the most important, is vanity. The average overweight person is awkward. Of course! Who wouldn't be awkward, with ten or twenty or fifty superfluous pounds strapped around his body! The average fat person does not look well in his—or her— clothes. You have to wear large sizes, so that, to begin with, the cut is not too youthful, and the result is a shapeless bag, more than likely. Three years ago, I found myself going from size 18 to size 20. The size 20 dresses had no style. They required a lot of alteration. And after they were altered I still looked like what I was—a short, squat woman with a bad figure. I lost twenty-five pounds. Now I wear a size 12 dress. Because I'm short (I couldn't do anything about that) I have to have hems turned up two inches—but that's the only alteration necessary. And for the first time in years I get compliments on my figure. I weigh no, but my bones are small, so I'm not thin. But I'm no longer a tub, thank you!

But it isn't just vanity that makes weight important. It's health, most of all.

Your weight has a definite bearing on how long you are likely to live. Persons who weigh too much have a far greater mortality, physicians have proved, than people of normal weight. Dr. Louis I. Dublin, Statistician of the Metropolitan Life Insurance Company, in an article in *Human Biology,* entitled "The Influence of Weight on Certain Causes of Death," shows, through a study of 200,000 cases, how dangerous overweight can be. The death rate for men and women of normal weight is 844 per 100,000. In the overweight group, the rate jumps to 1,111 per 100,000. In other words, the fat person has an excess mortality of from 14%, if you're very young, to as high as 86%, as you grow older.

You don't want to die! Of course not! Being alive can be a lot of fun. Well, the overweight person shows up pretty badly in all of Dr. Dublin's findings. Overweight folks constantly jeopardize their chances for a long life. Fat people practically commit suicide! They die by their own fat. An exaggeration? Just look at the statistics. Deaths from cardiovascular diseases are 62% above average for the too-fat population. Diabetes claims 167% above normal—yes, 167%—that's not a typographical error. In cancer, only 10% above average is the rate of death of the overweight—but even that is something to think about. 12% above average is the fat person's rate for accidental deaths. Fat people move and think a bit more slowly in emergencies, you see.

Have I frightened you? Well, that's what I've tried to do. In fact, I mention the very worst first of all, to jolt you into seeing the seriousness of too much fat. But, of course, you are not going to die because you're overweight! You're sure of that! Even so, it is just possible that you may become ill because you weigh too much. I don't mean that diseases are always brought about because of overweight. I do mean that you have a better chance of living longer if you are slim, and your health— the health of everyone—can be improved by the correction and prevention of obesity.

Some of the diseases on which obesity has an adverse influence are hypertension—high blood pressure to you— pulmonary emphysema, diabetes, various forms of heart disease, cancer, acute and chronic nephritis, venous thrombosis and embolism and arteriosclerosis. In pregnancy, the obese woman is susceptible to various types of illness. Many other diseases may be ameliorated to a great (degree by treating overweight—diseases for which, up until now, no actually successful treatment has been found.

Operations are far more dangerous if the patient is overweight. Doesn't it stand to reason that it is dangerous to cut through fat—which does not heal as quickly nor as well as healthy, non-fat tissue? In their excellent book, *Obesity,* Dr. Edward H. Rynearson and Dr. Clifford F. Gastineau, of the Mayo Clinic, both obesity experts, show the dangers of overweight and give many rules for getting back to normal.

Dr. John Joseph Lalli, whose specialty is arthritis, wrote me about overweight:

"In the city of New York alone, there are approximately 12,000 people in whom chronic arthritis has reached maturity in complete or partial ankylosis. Of greatest importance is the prevention of those particular manifestations which result in deformities. The unhealthy soil in which the seed of disease readily grows argues for early use of systematic methods of treatment before the joint segments or adjacent muscles and tendons are affected. The onset, manifested by painful soft-tissue swelling, as in atrophic-rheumatoid arthritis, can be successfully combated. In this disease, prevention is better than cure. Hypertrophic osteoarthritis, due mainly to the wear and tear of life, is also a problem of prevention. *Overweight, when present, may be likened to a wagonload of stones being drawn up a hill by a horse. The load is too heavy for the horse to pull. Either the horse must be whipped or the load lightened.* Often overweight breaks down the metatarsal arches, causing them to become flat and painful, with accompanying backache and other forerunners of chronic arthritis. In both types, systematic manifestations such as abnormal weight, nervousness, restlessness and excitability, loss of mental vigor, neuritic sensations, varying pulse rate, constipation, muscle atrophy, flat feet, nervous twitchings at night and general weakness are present."

Drs. Rynearson and Gastineau feel that other illnesses may be caused by, or exaggerated by, obesity, increased incidence of gallbladder disease, earlier appearance of varicose veins, more frequent fractures, increased fetal mortality and greater difficulty in obstetrical delivery are further reasons for the correction of obesity. It is probable that obesity increases the chances of development of both hypertension and diabetes. It has been suggested that since one action of insulin is to convert carbohydrates to fat, a process of considerable magnitude in the development of obesity, the demand for insulin is correspondingly great and may exceed the capacity of the pancreas to produce it; thus diabetes may result."

Drs. H. L. Smith and F. A. Willius, writing on "Adoposity of the Heart," show that cardiac enlargement in obesity is proportional to the increase in surface area, and that some of these otherwise normal enlarged hearts may fail. So—if you're fat, the fat around your heart may cause serious trouble. Or fatty infiltration—droplets of fat—may appear within the cardiac muscle cells.

But even that isn't all. Obesity may cause a diminished capacity for breathing because of restricted respiratory movements caused by deposits in the abdominal and thoracic walls. You should be able to breathe deeply, for health.

I could quote dozens of other authorities. But their findings all boil down to the same essential facts. Obesity can actually cause serious diseases. It can cause other diseases to become more serious. It is, in itself, a disease. And the longer a person is too fat, the harder it is to overcome the damage that the fat has done.

You wouldn't knowingly eat poison if you knew that the poison would hurt your system—and perhaps kill you. You wouldn't carry around a huge lead weight, if the weight were unbecoming, tiresome and dangerous—and kept your lungs from functioning properly, your heart from beating the way it should. You wouldn't want to have high blood pressure, arthritis, gout, a dozen other ills that obesity can cause or encourage. You surely would go out of your way to avoid, rather than bring about, diabetes.

This is the unpleasant part of what I have to tell you. I wanted to tell it to you first, not so you can forget it—because I don't want you to do that—but so you can realize how serious obesity really is. It isn't just something that keeps you from being attractive—though it may do that, too. It's a very serious disease—and you have it in your power to get rid of it.

Why not avoid serious illness, if you can avoid it—get rid of a burden that can only be an annoyance ?

Are you satisfied that being slender is the only course for you ? Good! Then you're really on the road to thinking yourself thin.

CHAPTER 2

Live long
and like it

IF YOU'VE BEEN THINKING about all the horrible things
that can—and easily might—happen to you if you are
fat, I'm sure you've decided to become thin. And to
live a long and, I hope, contented and useful life. Ready
to think yourself thin?

You realize, of course, that, like all other seemingly
easy things, there's a catch to it. Yes, you're going to
think yours. If thin. But you're going to do a lot of other
things besides. Thinking is part of it—a big part. But
you've got to do a great deal more than just sit and
think. Your telephone, the chair you're sitting in, the
clothes you're wearing, these words that you're reading—
they were all thoughts, first of all. But the thoughts
were translated into action before they became material
things. So your thoughts about getting thin, if you really
want to be thin, will have to be translated into action, too.
And the result will be you—the way you'd like to be.

You'll have to make yourself over! Your overweight
has been caused by wrong thinking—by a wrong way
of life—for you. The same way of life might not have
caused overweight for a lot of other people but, face

it, it has caused overweight for you. That means that it is wrong for you. So you must acquire a new viewpoint, an entire new outlook. And with this new outlook you must follow through until you look—and are—the person you'd like to be.

You know dozens of people, as I do, who have started diets, and never finished them. They've been enthusiastic, and lost ten pounds, or eighteen pounds. And then, within a few weeks, gained all of the pounds back again—and maybe added a few more for good measure. I know one man who did even better—or worse—than that. He went to an expensive doctor, who examined him and gave him a diet.

"Have you started your diet?" I asked him.

"No," he said. "I'm going away for a five-day weekend. When I come back I'll start."

I talked to him two weeks later.

"How is your diet going?" I asked.

"Oh, I haven't started yet," he told me. "You see, it's very difficult for me to diet because I'm not too well. In fact, I must have an operation, but the doctor doesn't want to operate until I lose weight. But I have to sort of work myself up to get into the mood to diet. I'll begin any day, now."

He hasn't started yet. But then he weighs only 233 pounds! The poor dear looks like a football, never feels well, and is still suffering from an injury to his leg, which happened three years ago, because his weight keeps it from healing properly. He'll never get thin until he learns about obesity—and he refuses to learn.

In the last analysis, you're all you have. Your family, your friends, even your earthly possessions, are yours in a far less realistic way. You can do a lot about developing your mind and your soul. But without a good body, your mind and your soul, things being what they are on this earth, will be in a pretty difficult spot. To become thin, in the way you should be thin, you must learn to have a disciplined mind, to be a responsible person. Instead of rationalizing your indulgences, you must realize your potentialities. You have the opportunities for discipline and, though the word may seem out of place here, for culture. You can become physically and mentally the person you should be only by putting thought to it.

Now you can't get thin unless you understand your body. And your mind, too. Otherwise you can dip into fifty diets. Some will reduce you. Others will leave you about where you were. Some will be helpful. Others might not be so good. But there will be no permanent change unless you know where you're going, and know what to do about it. You may get on a bus and ride and ride. It may be most interesting along the way. But unless you know where you want to go, and take the bus that will get you there, at the end you won't be much better off than you were when you started. Good luck *may* land you at your destination, but it isn't at all likely. Usually, you'll be worn out, far from home, and a little mystified because things happened the way they did. Any good diet will reduce you. But unless you learn about obesity, and learn why you, yourself, are fat, and then

apply the right remedy for you, you won't reduce properly—and you won't stay thin.

Staying thin, you know, is as important as getting thin.
No use getting thin, having all of your clothes made over,
and being proud of your figure and your appearance, if you
don't understand the principles underlying it—and get fat
again.

The new way of life which you must adopt, if you wish to
get thin and stay that way, must be different for you— and
once you've started it, you must keep up forever.

There are two schools of thought on losing weight. One
says that you must do it in secret—or talk about it only
with people who are reducing too. A sort of fat peoples'
Alcoholics Anonymous. In fact, there have been a lot of
attempts to start societies called Fatties Anonymous and
Gluttons Anonymous and Dieters Anonymous. I don't
believe in secret dieting. And I don't think you need any sort
of "Anonymous" society. I think that you should tell people
that you are trying to lose weight. Simplest thing in the
world! Saves a lot of annoyance, too. Hollywood stars
don't mind admitting that they are on diets—and most of
them are, because everyone knows that it is their business to
keep their figures trim. Isn't it your business, too? You needn't
keep the entire conversation buzzing around your figure or your
diet. Eat and drink the things you should eat and drink.
Whenever anything is offered that you should not have,
don't accept it and then waste it or mince it on your plate—
eating a bit too much the while. Just smile and say, "I'm
sorry I must refuse—that's not on my diet." Smile when

you say it—and don't weaken! And be as strict with yourself when you're alone as you are when company is around. Remember that the things you eat in secret between meals are every bit as fattening as the things you order in restaurants or have on your plate at dinner. The subject of obesity has always been a fascinating one. Early stone statues show that in 2,000 B.C. fat women were considered most desirable. They were popular, too, in savage tribes. The fact that they didn't live very long didn't seem to make much difference. The life span of the warriors of the tribe wasn't a great deal longer. By the time the Greeks began to find out what civilization and culture were really about, the wise men had begun to find out about obesity, too. Hippocrates, the father of modern medicine, found out that fat people were far more apt to die suddenly than were thin ones. Galen, too, was against obesity, and when he discovered that fevers reduced weight, he even thought it might be a good idea to induce fevers as weight reducers. In Greece and Rome, obesity was desirable—for their enemies, and Roman horsemen actually forfeited their horses if they gained too much weight.

In Elizabethan times, obesity was frowned upon. And Shakespeare, who introduced abnormal psychology quite a while before the modern boys thought of it—a sort of a pre-dated Freud—wrote,

"Make less thy body hence, and more thy grace,
Leave gormandizing; know the grave doth gape
For thee thrice wider than for other men."

There have been, of course, famous fat men through the ages, but they have been the exceptions. Chesterfield wrote, "Obesity and stupidity are such constant companions that they are considered synonymous." Napoleon grew fat only as he grew older—after his retreat from Moscow.

Our modern therapy for obesity was initiated in 1863. A man named William Banting started it. He was an undertaker, and, when his weight reached 200 pounds, he consulted an English doctor, William Harvey, because his hearing was affected. Banting was put on a diet which did not allow carbohydrates or fats. Banting gave up bread and butter, sugar, potatoes, beans and beer. His water intake was limited. On rye bread and meat and a few other things, he lost nearly fifty pounds. He wrote a book about it—and to this day a lot of folks talk about "Banting" when they mean dieting.

In Victoria's day, a plump woman with a well-rounded figure was considered quite an eyeful. And even here in America, at the turn of the Century and later, the well-developed actress was the one who received the most admiration. In *A Pictorial History Of The American Theatre,* by Daniel Blum, which covers a fifty-year period, starting in 1900, the illustrations show that the actors and actresses of earlier times had figures which to-day would cause obesity specialists to start writing prescriptions immediately. James O'Neill, Delia Fox, Marie Cahill, May Irwin, Lillian Russell and Ada Rehan were all too fat, by modern standards. On the other hand, Fritzi Scheff, Nance O'Neill, Lionel Barrymore, Grace

George, Evelyn Nesbit, Blanche Sweet and Ethel Barrymore were all quite slender in their youth, and the fact that they are alive as I write might well be the result of their lack of fat.

During the Flapper Twenties, the thin girl came into her own. Reproductions of John Held's drawings—typical of the period in their smooth sophistication—show flat-chested, small-waisted girls, living rapidly, if not too wisely.

The thin girl stayed in fashion for a long time. During the years waists stayed small, but breasts began to be fuller and more rounded. Today, with the help of New York nightclub columnist Earl Wilson, and such actresses as Miss Russell—Jane, not Lillian—the rounded figure is in fashion, once more.

The modern girl has gained weight—but she is not fat. Her waist and hips are small. Her back is straight. Statistics show that the average woman is only 5 feet 4 inches in height, and not too slender, but today's girls are thin enough, physically. They are mentally well-balanced. And they are healthy, too.

The professional model is today's ideal, as far as figures are concerned. For style and distinction, she takes the place of the chorus girl of two generations ago, and the show girl of the last generation. Recently, while writing a series of articles for the Hearst Publications' King Features, I interviewed some of New York's most successful models. One at a time, a dozen of these girls, with their hat boxes—practically a symbol of their profession—came to my apartment. I asked them questions about themselves.

Today's models are tall, I found out from these girls, and from studying the descriptions of dozens of other models. The average height ranges from five feet seven inches to five feet nine inches—in high heels. Quite a bit taller than Miss or Mrs. Average American. Their weights vary—weight isn't too important, for the girls realize that bone structure causes a great weight variation. Most of the girls weighed around one hundred and twenty-five pounds.

Model sizes didn't vary a great deal. Most of the successful models, I discovered, have busts which measure thirty-four inches, waists twenty-four inches, and hips thirty-four inches—or the same as the bust measurement. These girls usually wear size 12 dresses—the "model" size—though size 10 can also be worn. The Junior "model" size is one inch less in waist, hips and bust. You may not be as tall as a model, but it would be very nice, unless you're a great big girl, if you managed to get down to model size in most of your dimensions.

Male models, though they do not set the fashions, as the feminine models do, still have excellent figures that could serve as ideal for the male population. Most of them are tall—around six feet—but there are a number of successful male models who are only five feet ten inches tall. The average male model wears a 15½-inch shirt and has a waist that measures 31 inches. I don't say that all men should have those measurements, but both male and female models from the Conover Agency or the

Society of Models do manage to stay slim, attractive looking and healthy.

Before you write to me and accuse me of trying to turn all American men and women into professional models—in size, anyhow—I want to tell you that I don't want, expect or advise you to become this slender. I'm not even dangling this carrot of perfection in front of your noses, except to say how pleasant it would be. I am trying to show you how the average figure has changed through the years—and that our present ideal, as shown by the clothes horses who display, professionally, modern clothes, is a slim but pleasantly rounded young woman, or a slim, flat-stomached, broad-shouldered young man.

Life expectancy has increased, during the years, from a potential twenty-three years in Rome to thirty-five years during the Renaissance—with a far shorter life expectancy in the ages before that. In 1900, life expectancy was fifty years, and present life expectancy is sixty-four years for men and seventy years for women. Only fat people have a shorter life expectancy—almost one per cent less for each pound of superfluous flesh—20% less for the man or woman who is 20% overweight, and far more than that for the really fat man or woman. I refuse to look again at the figures for the men and women who carry around a burden of over fifty pounds of excess blubber.

You needn't look like a model. You should look like yourself—your better self, the self that you could be, once your body has sloughed off needless and useless fat. You'll live longer, and have more fun living, too, once your weight has reached normal for your height. Once you've learned to think yourself thin.

What can you do about it? Well, to begin with, here are my first directions: Please order, at once, two good sets of scales. One set is for your bathroom. I prefer the Borg Scale or the Detecto doctor's type scale. Why? Because those scales have readable numbers, and are usually reliable.

I might as well tell you right now that I expect to mention a great many manufactured articles by name— and that none of the firms is paying me a cent for the publicity— or even knows that I'm mentioning them. I don't own a single share of stock in any of the firms who manufacture any articles of apparel, food or kitchen utensils. I wish I did 1 I've refused a commercial offer for the recipe for Magicream—my imitation whipped cream, which you'll learn how to make, later on—so I could give it to you, for free. I'm mentioning things by name not so much to please the manufacturers, though I feel they will be pleased, as to help you get the things that much experimenting has shown me are the most satisfactory.

For the second scales, get a good set for your kitchen. But don't get kitchen scales, because most of them, though fairly accurate, are so arranged that they weigh merchandize up to twenty-five pounds, and while they are fine for weighing fairly heavy purchases of groceries, they are not good for weighing small amounts in ounces— and that is what you'll use them for. You might buy a medical scale, which is expensive, and completely accurate. Or, if money is an object, you'll be satisfied, I'm sure, with a good letter scale, which is not expensive, and can be used for your mail, too. The Hanson scale is a good one, and weighs accurately, by ounces, up to two pounds—and I'm sure you'll not want to weigh anything more than that amount.

Most weight reducing authorities have a definite rule about weighing—yourself and not your food. They believe in weighing once a week—or every two or three weeks. Personally, I go mad if I can't weigh myself every day! Last year, while traveling abroad, I breathed a great sigh of satisfaction when I was a guest at the home of Ambassador and Mrs. Avra Warren, and found, in their bathroom, an accurate scale. The satisfaction of weighing myself almost made up for the fact that I'd gained five pounds.

You certainly don't have to weigh all of the food you eat. Occasionally, you'll have to weigh portions of food, so you might as well have the scales handy in the kitchen. But I do heartily approve of weighing yourself every day in your own bathroom. I know one fat man who said he wanted to reduce, but who told me that his bathroom scales wouldn't work very well.

"Why don't you buy a new one?" I asked.

"I can't afford it," he told me. And proceeded to spend large sums of money on entertaining guests at dinners and cocktails. He lost *ten* pounds, he told me, but he couldn't be sure. That inaccurate scale, you see!

He's continued to be fat—and doesn't want to know what he weighs.

If you want to get thin—and I hope you do—please get those two scales right away. And use the bathroom scales every day.

The best—and most optimistic—time to weigh yourself is in the morning, after you've "wrung yourself out." Weigh yourself in the nude, wearing only bedroom slippers. If you weigh yourself every morning at just about the same time, you'll get a pretty accurate idea of your weight. As you begin reducing, make a note of this weight every day. Even if the scale does not show a daily reduction, because of food you've eaten the day before that may have been bulky, even if not fattening, the daily weighing is the most satisfactory way you have of finding out how you are getting along toward reaching your ideal weight and size.

More directions—and these must be followed if you intend to lose weight according to this Think Yourself Thin method—and I hope you do. Buy a small note book. No, don't use loose sheets of paper and tell yourself they'll be just as good. They won't be! You're going to analyze yourself in a number of ways. The note book is essential. It may be lined or unlined—it's up to you to choose the kind that is most convenient. It shouldn't be too small in size. It should be one that can be tucked into a drawer that is near your bed. The ideal place to keep it is in your bed table drawer, but any drawer that has a bit of room in it will do.

Now, starting today—or tomorrow if that is more

convenient for you, but certainly not a minute later— write down every single thing you eat, with the amount of it, as nearly as you can estimate, in cupfuls or half-cupfuls. This need not be absolutely accurate as to measurements. It should be accurate as to foods. Write down what you eat for breakfast. Draw a line. Then all of the foods or drinks you have in between. Write down the number of glasses or cups of liquids you consume— water, tea, coffee, milk. The first day or two you'll probably forget a number of things. Train yourself to think accurately—to remember. You'll need these pages for reference later on, so keep them as neatly and as accurately as you can. Child's play? No, indeed. Only by a recording of the foods you eat can you arrive at any conclusion about your food and liquid intake. You must find out why you're fat before you can be cured permanently.

Don't say, "It isn't the food. I eat like a bird," and let it go at that. If you are too fat, then you eat too much. That's the basic truth. FOOD MAKES FAT!

Of course, you know that some people do not get fat, no matter how much they eat. We all know of lucky people who can gobble the most fattening viands and gain not a single ounce. I know a lovely young girl with a waist so slender a man can—and does—span it easily with his two hands, and she devours mounds of rich desserts, great fluffs of whipped cream, huge portions of chocolate pie. Disgusting—if you're fat, and can't imitate her. On the other hand, I've known fat people who can gain seven pounds over a week-end of fairly rich living, and not lose an ounce of it when the week-end is over. Food makes fat——-and it makes fat more quickly for some folks than for others. It's up to you to find out why it is making fat for you—to regulate the causes, if possible, and otherwise to regulate the results.

You'll have to diet, of course. But, if you find out why you are fat, and correct the "why," the results may be far better than you have any reason to expect. There may be purely physical reasons for your overweight. There may be psychosomatic reasons—a combination of body and mind. Or the reasons may be purely mental. Once you know the real cause of your overweight, it is far easier to get to the results. Even your dieting will be far less annoying—and much more rewarding. And diets aren't half bad, anyhow, when you've learned what to eat, and how to order or prepare it. It's the tasteless and monotonous diet, that does not satisfy your hunger, which is bad. You won't have to have that at all. Your diet can be fairly exciting, even if it is strict. And it may not even have to be strict. Of this much, however, I'm sure—if you are overweight you will have to change your eating habits, and your habits of thought about food. Food makes fat. You are what you eat. Those two facts are inseparable. The badly adjusted fat person can gain weight on food that would leave a thin person practically starving. When you've learned to change your food habits, and your food thoughts, you'll grow slender. And you'll stay that way, though you never again can slip back into your old ways of eating and thinking.

So, to think yourself thin, buy the two sets of scales,

unless you have them already. And don't tell me—or yourself—that the old, inaccurate ones will do. They won't do at all! Accurate scales are your first "must" for reduction. The note book is the second. They are your first necessities. You are taking the first steps to thinking yourself thin.

CHAPTER 3

The weigh of
all flesh

WHEN ARE YOU GOING TO BEGIN TO REDUCE? Don't get impatient about it! Sit back and relax—and learn about yourself. When you've learned the principles of sensible living for you, then you can begin to lose weight.

After all, you've probably been overweight for a long time. You're not going to lose weight suddenly, anyhow. In fact, there is no way to lose a lot of weight at one time that is not dangerous to health. Another thing— weight lost rapidly, unless you understand the underlying reasons, comes back just as quickly. When you become slender I want you to stay that way. It's a job, a whole new way of living. But I think you'll find it is worth it. I hope so, anyhow. A firm, slender, healthy body, a youthful face, for your age, and a sensible outlook on living—aren't those things worth waiting for?

In the meantime, you are disciplining yourself. You are weighing yourself every morning, after you've attended to your toilet, in the nude and wearing only bedroom slippers. Mark down this weight. It may not vary very much from day to day, but it will give you the habit of weighing yourself. And it will give you tables for

24

comparison, as you grow more slender. And, in the note book I asked you to get, you are writing down everything you eat, and, if possible, the times you ate it. This should be done the last thing at night. Discipline and training again, but, far more important, another list that will prove valuable when you start to reduce. These are the first two "musts" on your program. And don't write to me a month from now and tell me that you wrote down a couple of days' weight and a couple of days' menus, but that you got bored and quit. You can reduce by my method only if you write down these two things every day: your weight in the morning, and the day's complete food—and drink—intake at night.

You want to be normal, I'm sure. Normal in health and weight. But what is normal? We must accept statistics for that, unless we have the time and the money to gather our own facts—and I don't know who has. Normality isn't necessarily the 34-24-34-inch slenderness of the average professional female model, nor the 15½-inch shirt, 31-inch waist of the professional male model. Nor is it even the measurements from "Women's Measurements for Garment and Pattern Construction," developed by the United States Department of Agriculture for the manufacturers of America, which shows the average woman is 5 feet 4 inches in height, and weighs more than 130 pounds. You see, the twenty-odd millions of women who are too fat have influenced these results. These charts show the way women are, not the way they should be.

How fat *should* one be? Obesity, according to medical

authorities, is the condition of the body in which the weight, because of excessive storage of fat, is above normal. People who are from ten to fifteen per cent above normal are considered just slightly fat. Those who are more than fifteen per cent above normal are really obese. According to Ebstein, the classifications of fat people are: "Those who inspire envy, those who provoke laughter and those who call forth sympathy." Dr. James S. McLester, Professor of Medicine at the University of Alabama, in his excellent book, *Nutrition And Diet In Health And Disease,* divides obesity into two divisions: simple obesity, which includes alimentary, or exogenous; and constitutional, or endogenous, and the obesity which accompanies other disorders, and includes the glandular types, pituitary, gonad, adrenal cortex and thyroid.

What does this mean? Simple   enough, actually. Alimentary obesity results from the indulgence of appetite, plus a good digestion. In other words, eating too much makes fat. Food makes fat! The normal person—the one who can eat a lot without gaining weight—probably has within his own body some form of regulatory mechanism which balances appetite against physical activity. He maintains body weight by eating exactly the amount that the body can take care of. However, the person who has alimentary obesity is not this fortunate. His mechanism does not work, does not synchronize properly. So the person with this trouble eats too much or moves around too little—uses up too little energy— so, for him, his intake of food is too great, and the part that is not used up in energy is stored as fat. The amount of food which would seem to be right and appropriate proves too great, at least for the amount of energy used. We'll go into details about the reasons for this, later on.

Constitutional obesity is thought by experts to be the result of faulty metabolism or some other physical aberration which causes the accumulation of fat. A lowered basal metabolism or an incorrect water balance may cause the accumulation of fat. We'll go into all this in detail, later, too. Now we're interested only in establishing what may be considered normal. The normal person, then, is one whose system—including digestion, glands, water balance and mental and emotional stability—is such that the amount of food eaten is exactly balanced by bodily activities. In other words, the person who is normal weighs exactly what he should, according to his height and bone structure—and he eats exactly the amount necessary for his way of life to maintain the weight. Thus, a man of normal weight doing heavy physical exercise will use up a certain amount of food—an amount that will be just right for him. The same man eating the same amount of food, if he doesn't work so hard, would get fat. But if he is normal, he has a normal appetite and will eat only what he needs, so when he works less, he eats less. In other words, the mechanics of his body are perfect. Granting that he can get the food he wants and needs, he chooses just enough to maintain his body at the correct weight.

The fat person, on the other hand, either has an ungovernable appetite, and eats more than he needs, or his bodily mechanism is so slow that he doesn't use up the food. Think of the body as a furnace. The properly balanced furnace, if given the right kind and amount of fuel, will burn brightly, and use up practically all the fuel, with only the average amount of residue, which will pass from the body. The furnace that is not in proper working order will burn slowly or faultily. The food will not be consumed properly. Food—and water, too—will be kept within the body, to add unnecessary weight. Of course, we are living creatures and not furnaces, so the analogy is not perfect. However, one thing is absolutely certain. If you are too fat, you are eating too much food for you. It may not be too much for other people—even people of your exact height, build and circumstance. It may not be too much for you, once your system is in good condition. Or it may be the wrong kind of food—incorrectly balanced. But, if you are overweight right now, you are eating too much food—for you. Food makes fat. I hope you'll learn why you're fat and how you're fat and where you're fat—and how to do something about it, before too long.

This is about the normal person—that ideal creature who eats as much as he feels like eating and doesn't gain a pound, but stays at the weight at which nature intended him to be. Now, there are several points about this normal person that seem to be hazy to the average person—even if he is over or underweight. First of all, there is no such thing as a "normally fat man" or a "normally fat woman." I've even heard experts talk of "normally fat" patients, whom they wouldn't think of reducing. A person may come from a family of fat people. He may have been born fat, and, because of family conditions, kept too fat all of his life, but he's still a fat person and not "normally fat" at all. He may well have a tendency toward corpulency. But he's not normally fat. In fact, he can be reduced, just the same as anyone else, without injuring health or appearance, and look and feel better. Then he'll be a normal person in weight, and not at all "normally fat." If you are too fat then you should reduce until your weight is right—normal—for you. Then you should maintain that weight. It may, and probably will, mean a whole change of your routine of living, your plans, even your outlook on life. From what I've seen, I think it will be an improvement.

I know a lot of fat people who are delightful. They are wonderful companions, quick witted, kind, pleasant. But they are still too fat. And they'd get more pleasure out of life, and have a better chance of enjoying more years of life, if they were slender. They are getting along just fine. I love them the way they are. But I can't help wishing they were a little nearer weight perfection.

How much food does the normal person require? It seems excessive to the fat person, who can eat only a part of that amount. And the worst of it is that, even when your weight has reached perfection, you probably can't eat as much as these lucky individuals, who don't even have to know anything about calories or weight reduction. But you should know these amounts so you can compare them with your requirements and intake.

Physicians have estimated the following requirements for the maintenance of weight by the normal person. You'll see by consulting your calorie tables—and a lot more about them, later—how very liberal this allowance seems. It would be nice if my wand were in order, so I could wave it and wish that we could all eat these generous amounts and not gain an ounce.

Occupation	Calorie Requirement Per Day
Housework, light	1,500 to 2,000
Seamstress	1,500 to 2,000
Typist	1,500 to 2,500
Salesgirl	1,500 to 2,500
Housework, heavy	2,000 to 2,500
Clerk	2,000 to 3,000
Business Executive	2,200 to 3,000
Outside Salesman	2,300 to 3,000
Dancer	3,000 to 3,500
Heavy Labor	4,500 to 5,300

How much should you weigh, once you have got back to your normal weight? There are a lot of opinions about that, too. It used to be thought that a person should grow heavier as he grew older—and most of the old-fashioned tables show this—with only very old people losing a little. I'm not going to show you these obsolete tables, even for comparison. It is now accepted by practically all good authorities that people should not grow heavier as they grow older. The experts have found that the most efficient and successful men and women are those who attain their right weight around their twenty-fifth or twenty-sixth year, although they may keep on gaining a very little until they reach thirty. This should be their ideal weight, and should be maintained easily through the years.

The best weight tables are those devised by the Metropolitan Life Insurance Company. These are based on numerous Medico-Actuarial studies of hundred of thousands of insured men and women. They are reproduced here on page 34. Find your own height by the simple method of standing up against a wall, and asking someone to take a ruler, put it on your head, and mark your height on the wall. Then measure the mark. When you've found your size on the tables, you'll have found your perfect weight. You'll have to decide for yourself whether your bony frame is small, medium or large. But anyone who has even minimum powers of observation ought to be able to decide which category he belongs in. My wrists and ankles are small, my bones are thin. So, naturally, it follows that I have a small frame and should weigh the smallest amount for my height. You see, too, every frame size has a variation, so that each height has an allowable variance of about fifteen pounds.

Choose your ideal weight. But don't cheat! Don't fool yourself. If you are small boned, don't pick out the largest amount for your height, by telling yourself that your bones are large. And if your bones are large, don't go to the other extreme and become discouraged because you tell yourself that you must lose the maximum amount. Be fair. And decide on your perfect weight as soon as possible. You can do that, with these tables, as well as any expert.

Once you've found your perfect weight, you'll know how much you'll have to lose. And you'll know the weight you should maintain all of the rest of your life.

Decided how much you have to lose? Now all you need think about, until you take the next step, is how much time you should take to reach the perfect weight for you. How much should you reduce each week? The fatter you are, the more you can lose. If you are extremely fat, you may safely lose four or even five pounds a week, at the beginning, with a steady loss of two or three pounds a week after that. If you are a hundred pounds overweight, you can count on reaching your perfect weight in about a year. Most people are lucky in that they do not have to lose such a huge amount of superfluous fat.

If your weight is only fifteen or twenty-five—or even forty—pounds above what it ought to be, then your task ahead is much simpler. You might lose three pounds a a week for the first few weeks, then two pounds a week for a week or two, and then one pound a week until your ideal weight has been reached. With the necessary "rests" in between, it may take you six months to reach the weight you'd like to have—and keep. But it undoubtedly took you much longer to gain all of that weight. If you lose weight slowly, your skin will look better, and, with proper care, you won't have any reduction wrinkles, your muscles will be strong and supple, and you won't feel tired or weak. The result, all around, will be better—

physically and psychologically. Of course, if there were only some magical way to get slender overnight it would be much better—but I've never heard of that being accomplished, even in fiction. I have heard of spectacular losses but some of them were followed by loss of health, and none was permanent. Become slender gradually— and stay that way.

Desirable Weights for Men and Women of Ages 25 and Over
Weight in Founds According to Frame   (as Ordinarily Dressed)

MEN

HEIGHT (with shoes on) Feet Inches	SMALL FRAME	MEDIUM FRAME	LARGE FRAME
5 2	116–125	124–133	131–142
3	119–128	127–136	133–144
5 4	122–132	130–140	137–149
5	126–136	134–144	141–153
5 6	129–139	137–147	145–157
7	133–143	141–151	149–162
5 8	136–147	145–156	153–166
9	140–151	149–160	157–170
5 10	144–155	153–164	161–175
11	148–159	157–168	165–180
5 0	152–164	161–173	169–185
1	157–169	166–178	174–190
5 2	163–175	171–184	179–196
3	168–180	176–189	184–202

WOMEN

HEIGHT (with shoes on —1½" heel) Feet Inches	SMALL FRAME	MEDIUM	LARGE FRAME
4 11	104—111	110—118	117—127
0	105—113	112—120	119—129
5	107—115	114—122	121—131
1	110—118	117—125	124—135
5	113—121	120—128	127—138
2	116—125	124—132	131—142
5	119—128	127—135	133—145
3	123—132	130—140	138—150
5	126—136	134—144	142—154
4	129—139	137—147	145—158
5	133—143	141—151	*149—162*
5	136—147	145—155	*152—166*
5	139—15Ò	148—158	*155—169*

These tables are reprinted here through the courtesy of the Metropolitan Life Insurance Company.

CHAPTER 4

Eat to live

THIS ISN'T A FUN BOOK. There have been dozens of books and articles written on weight reduction from the fun point of view. One of the best and most amusing —packed with good sense, too, and, of course, mighty well written—is *No Food With My Meals,* by Fannie Hurst, published by Harper. *The Fat Boy's Book,* by Elmer Wheeler, published by Prentice Hall, is amusing— and contains a lot of good information about losing weight, too·

This book is serious. I'm writing it under the supervision of a physician who is a specialist, with advice from another specialist, and with the books of dozens of recognized authorities as reference. Oh, I have some goodies tucked away toward the end—recipes that I worked out by myself—but you're not to look at them, now. You see, I'm working on a definite plan. Here is what it is: I believe, if you understand the subject of obesity, and understand yourself, that you'll use your brains and initiative and think yourself into the mood for getting thin. More than that, your thought will have some substance. You'll know what you're thinking about î So you'll have a new pattern of life, which will be the right pattern for you. It may not, and probably will not, be the comfortable pattern of eating and drinking rich things any time you want them, of slouching, or wasting yourself—and time. But you'll look better and feel better, you'll enjoy life more— and I actually believe you'll have more time left to enjoy it in.

So far, I hope you've learned some of the dangers of obesity. I've undoubtedly omitted a lot of them, but now you know the value of living sensibly, and the weight you should be to be healthy and happy. You know, too, how much weight you must lose. I hope you're establishing the habit of weighing yourself every morning and making notes of what you've eaten every night, for two reasons: To establish a routine, and to have a record for comparison and reference.

From now on, for quite a while, you'll be finding out what makes you the way you are—why you're too fat. And that covers many different angles, as you'll soon find out. Some of these you may know—undoubtedly will know, if you've been interested in getting thin for any length of time. Some of them may surprise you. But here they are, all together, in the order in which I think you'll find them most helpful.

Please read this book slowly, and in the order in which I've written it. If you read only one chapter a day—and the chapters are short—I'll be very much pleased. In three weeks you'll have read the whole book—and I believe you'll understand yourself a little better than you ever did before, and will be on the way to attaining the ideal figure for you.

Don't be annoyed if there are some repetitions! I've found out something. If I didn't repeat things you'd forget them or never take them seriously. This way—pounding them in, the way the advertising experts do—you may even remember and follow my directions!

How much do you actually know about your need for food and its utilization? Not too much, I'm afraid, after talking to a lot of folks who pose as experts. I wish I had a few hundred pages to spend on this subject. If you're interested, I can recommend some fine books for you. The best of the lot, it seems to me, is *Nutrition And Diet In Health And Disease,* by James S. Me-Lester, M.D., Professor of Medicine, University of Alabama, published by W. B. Saunders Co. I've referred to it before, and undoubtedly will again. Studying this book will give you a full course in nutrition. Good, too, for this part of your "learning" is *Diet And Personality,* by Dr. L. Jean Bogert, published by the Macmillan Co.

The Metropolitan Life Insurance Company, which is doing its full share in helping Americans realize the danger of overweight and in helping them to lose unneeded pounds, in cooperation with the United States Public Health Service and the American Medical Association, has devised an elaborate program on nutrition. Part of this work is concerned with group therapy. Two short movies, an eight-minute one, "Cheers for Chubby," and a twelve-minute one, "Losing to Win," will be seen this winter all over America. There is also a fine free booklet, "Overweight and Underweight," which the company will send you. I shall recommend other books that I've enjoyed, and that reputable physicians have recommended to me, as they pertain to what we're talking about.

Nutrition, as you well know, is the process by which living organisms receive and utilize materials necessary for maintaining life. This includes growth, repair and the supply of energy. Foodstuffs, made up mainly of carbohydrates, proteins and fats, contain energy which is liberated in the body. The actual energy can be measured in a test tube. The energy which food yields is expressed in units of heat know as calories. So, a calorie is the amount of heat energy necessary to raise the temperature of I kilogram of pure water from 15° to 16° F. Now, when you read about a calorie, you will know that it's only the energy needed to heat one tiny bit of water one degree. Not so mysterious, after all!

The usable part of this energy varies, of course. The following standard values have been generally adopted: One gram of carbohydrates yields 4.1 calories; one gram of protein, 4.1; and one gram of fat, 9.3. For ordinary purposes, the gram of carbohydrate yields 4 calories; the gram of protein, 4 calories; and the gram of fat, 9 calories.

Each of these foodstuffs has its own part to play. And right now you may as well realize that, in natural foods, you can't possibly eat one of these without eating some of the others. You may have a "high" protein diet or a "high" carbohydrate diet, but you can't completely eliminate any of them. Diets that tell you not to mix them are based on imagination more than fact.

Carbohydrates supply the energy that yields heat and

does mechanical work. They are the least expensive and the most easily obtainable source of muscle energy. But people who are poor and who must eat food that is almost all starch become too fat. That is why so many of our poorer people, even if they do hard work, grow extremely fat on a seemingly simple diet of bread, potatoes and other starchy vegetables, with perhaps beer as a beverage—and very little meat or other protein food.

Fats, on oxidation, liberate heat and contribute to the bodily warmth. They also furnish energy for muscular work. But you must realize, now, that each fat gram is over twice as heavy as his carbohydrate and protein brothers.

Proteins are the most expensive foodstuffs and experts are always wrangling over the amount needed for human health and maintenance. You'll find you need a lot of protein when you begin to reduce your weight. Proteins serve mainly to repair worn out tissues and to provide new tissues for growing organisms, but they may be converted into the same substances, and accomplish the same purposes, as carbohydrates and fats. All three are needed in the body. And when the body gets more than it needs, the rest is usually stored as fat. And we've completed the circle. Food makes fat!

Another group of food factors which are absolutely essential to health are the vitamins. Although unrelated chemically, they serve as part of the enzyme system, and each one exercises a distinct form of control over physiological processes.

Now, what happens to these foods when we eat them?

Digestion starts in the mouth. Saliva maintains the
water balance and actually aids digestion. Chewing helps,
too. The only pleasure we get from food is while it is
in our mouths—yet people who are fat invariably eat
too rapidly, do not chew their food well, and swallow
it before all of the flavors have been released. This is
odd, because fat people love to eat, and they are fat only
because, in the last analysis, they eat too much—for them.
Of course, there are exceptions. You probably do know
of a fat person who eats slowly and chews his food well,
and enjoys every mouthful of it to the last crumb. He
is unusual. The average fat person gobbles his food!

So, you are too fat. Here is your very first rule for
reduction—and you may not get another for a long
time, for you aren't ready for many rules, just now. Eat
slowly—much more slowly than you have been eating.
Chew each mouthful thoroughly. Do not swallow the
food until you've got all of the enjoyment out of it. I'm
not telling you to make yourself ridiculous or to "Fletch-
erize," and reduce your food to a liquid. I do say to
you: Take far smaller pieces. Cut your food into smaller
—much smaller—portions. Don't fill your fork or spoon.
Take a small bite. Pause a minute between bites, to en.
joy the flavor of your food. Chew each portion well.

Part of this same rule—or you may consider it a second
rule, if you like: Think about your food while you are
eating it. Enjoy it! The only way you can enjoy your
food is to think about its flavor and texture.

I know a man who got thin on this one rule alone.

'Td been gulping my food," he told me, "hardly

realizing what I was eating. I was amazed when I discovered what huge bites I was taking! I'd got into the habit of bad table manners because I'd had lunch with business acquaintances, who talked business and gulped their food. I ordered the first thing I thought of, whether I liked it or not. I was eating huge luncheons and dinners—and eating a lot of food I didn't even care for. When I began to think about what I ate, remembering to eat smaller bites and to chew my food well, I found that I ate much less—far smaller portions satisfied me. But that wasn't all! I began eating only the things I really liked. I became more particular in my choice of dishes. So unconsciously I discarded a lot of fattening foods. I was all ready to go on a strenuous diet—I was about forty pounds overweight in the beginning—when I found that I was already losing at just the rate I should lose. That's all I've done about eating. I do a few of the tightening exercises. My weight is down to normal, and I've never felt better. And I sure enjoy my meals a thousand times more! In fact, now I don't know what pleasure I ever got out of gulping down great hunks of meat and potatoes."

I don't promise that you'll get thin by this first rule. It certainly didn't reduce me much, though it did make me enjoy and appreciate food a lot more. But I know a good many people who haven't had to do a great deal more. For me, it was just a good start. That's what I hope it will prove for you, if it doesn't do more. Eat only the foods you enjoy—you're not on a diet—yet. Eat smaller bites. Chew each bite very well. Think about the flavors of the foods you are eating. You know that by will power you can think about practically anything that you wish. Unless you're in great physical discomfort, you should be the master of your own mind, and be able to think about anything you like. So think about your food, while you are eating it. Maybe you'd better watch your table manners, too. Like as not you've grown careless, without even knowing it. Do you grab your fork too near the tines, your knife handle too near the blade?

I don't mean that you're to become a bad dinner companion. Not at all! But you shouldn't talk with your mouth full, anyhow. The luncheon table and the dinner table are places for pleasant conversation. But you can talk and eat, too! Eating the food you like, and taking small bites—and thinking about it while you're eating it—is the first rule for getting thin. It's almost the first rule for good digestion. And it can become a very satisfactory rule for becoming a good dinner companion.

The digestive functions of the stomach, like the mouth, are mechanical and chemical. Food goes to the center of the stomach, where digestion is continued, and where the food remains alkaline. Then it is pushed toward the periphery, acid juices are worked into it, and it goes down toward the pylorus. In the stomach are pepsin and hydrochloric acid, which digest protein; rennin, which curdles milk; and a gastric juice which has a a lipolytic effect. Your digestion is influenced greatly by your mental state—in fact, a great percentage of stomach troubles are caused by worry or nerves, which affect the gastric juices.

One of the most unpleasant—and dangerous—ways of weight reduction is by expelling food from the stomach after it has been swallowed. A few years ago, it was considered not at all disgusting, by a group of young Hollywood actresses who wanted to lose weight. They excused themselves after eating—and forcibly ejected their dinners. They didn't even use an emetic. They just put their fingers down their throats. They felt that they had solved, though not too daintily, the problem of reducing. They preferred to eat large and rich meals, and then "upchuck" them immediately after dinner, to any other method of weight reduction.

There was just one trouble with their plan. It didn't work! One of the actresses died of cancer of the stomach. It was never thoroughly established that that was how she got a cancer of the stomach—and perhaps it wasn't. But she did die of cancer of the stomach, and she had had the habit of vomiting up her dinners immediately after eating them. Two more of the girls developed serious stomach trouble. The others felt they'd better stop their newfound habits.

In Rome, every fashionable home had its vomitorium. Several were discovered intact, elaborately built of carved marble, in the ruins of Pompeii. After a great feast or orgy, during which time the diners ate steadily for three or four hours, they would visit the vomitorium for the purpose of expelling all of the food they had eaten. The results seemed satisfactory at the time—but history doesn't bear this out. Rich Romans were old men at thirty-five, if they lived that long, and their life expectancy at birth, according to Dr. Martin Gumpert, was twenty-three years. Today it is sixty-seven for our whole population—higher for women than men—and is still higher for those of us who remain slender. So you see, the Roman use of the vomitorium had nothing to recommend it then—and it has less to recommend it today. After you've eaten, forget about your food and let nature take care of it. Your thoughts about food should be concerned about it before and during the meal.

The stomach becomes empty, after an ordinary meal, in from three to four-and-a-half hours. Your food will undoubtedly digest better if you do not drink water while you are eating. You'll reduce faster that way, too. I'll have a lot more to say about water later on.

From the stomach, the food goes into the small intestine, where muscular waves and chemicals continue the digestive processes. The pancreas and the liver help, too. In the large intestine, the formation of feces is completed. Many people believe that the feces consist of unabsorbed food residue. This isn't true. They consist of intestinal secretions and excretions of cellular material from intestinal walls, of bacteria, and only in small part of food residues. Concentrated foods, such as meat and cottage cheese, are absorbed to a great extent and leave little residue. Milk, bread, fruits and vegetables leave a large residue, mostly of indigestible cellulose. The composition and physical characteristics of the feces are determined, to a large extent, by what is eaten.

Frequently, when dieting, a light laxative is advised by a doctor, who knows the condition of his patient.

While a heavy purge is never advisable, a light laxative, which causes the food to pass more rapidly through the body, without being completely absorbed, often helps weight reduction without being injurious—when prescribed by a physician. Mineral oil is thought, by some authorities, to destroy vitamins. Other authorities think it is harmless. Mineral oil is not absorbed by the system in any way. It forms a coating to the intestines and helps the food slide by. It is completely tasteless. When recommended by physicians, it is often a valuable adjunct to diet, for the person who is allowed a small quantity of mineral oil can use it as a substitute for part of the olive oil in salad dressing, and, mixed with cooking oil, for cooking. Even frying with mineral oil is possible, and gives variation to a strict reducing diet. It should not be used without medical approval. Milk of magnesia, with medical approval, is often satisfactory, too.

I have described to you the nutritive elements, and what happens to food once it has gone into the system, because it seems to me that only by knowing your own body and what goes on in it can you become slender in anything resembling a scientific fashion. Only by understanding yourself can you think yourself thin.

CHAPTER 5

"It's my glands!"

IT'S ALWAYS A COMFORT for fat people to sit back and say, contentedly, "It's my glands, you know!" I'm sure you've heard dozens of fat people say exactly that. I know I have. And, curiously enough, maybe they are telling the truth—sometimes without actually realizing it.

Until recently, even experts were apt to disregard glandular disturbances as a cause of obesity. Now they admit that glands may have a lot to do with overweight— and they're doing something about it by prescribing proper treatment.

But even those whose obesity is glandular must realize one thing—that same old thing—food makes fat. The person with a glandular deficiency is still eating too much, and his overweight is still caused by overeating. Even with glandular correction he'll have to watch his diet, both during and after his treatment.

It is hard for a physician to say to a patient, "You're too fat because you're a glutton." Too often the patient comes back with, "Why Doctor, I eat hardly anything. I eat like a bird!"

46

Now, the physician can soften the blow by finding that perhaps the patient actually has some glandular disturbance. By treatment, plus a suitable diet, the patient loses weight a bit more easily. But it is still the diet that does it 1 Glandular treatment alone is seldom successful. Combined with diet it seemingly works miracles.

You don't believe that a glandular case can get thin even without treatment? You can prove it in no time at all. If any human being goes without food for a long enough period he will starve to death. And he'll get thin before he starves. So—a person who is too fat, for any cause in the world, can reduce his weight by simple starvation. Of course that is not the way to get thin for health. I'm mentioning this just to show you that glandular people can get thin if they go without eating. The proper treatment for a glandular case is proper medication plus a proper diet. It is only the fact that physicians now recognize glandular deficiencies as one cause of obesity that is new. Doctors were too apt to dismiss glandular cases as non-existent or unimportant, just a few years ago.

Glandular cases are still rare. And it is quite likely, if you are overweight—and you undoubtedly are, or you wouldn't be reading this far—that your trouble isn't glandular at all. There may be purely physical reasons why you are fat, or purely psychological reasons, or psychosomatic reasons. Physical, mental—or a combination of the two—those will probably contain the answer to your own personal too-fat condition. But you can't dismiss glands, without a serious consideration of them.

If you are interested in a more thorough study of glandular conditions than I can possibly give you here, there are three books that will prove valuable to you. They are: *Your Life Is In Your Glands,* by Herman H. Rubin, published by Stratford House; *Obesity,* by Dr. Edward H. Rynearson and Dr. Clifford F. Gastineau, published by Charles Thomas; and *The Management Of Obesity,* by Dr. Louis Pelner, published by Personal Diet Service.

But we can, even here, discuss the types of glandular obesity, so that you can tell, in a general way, if that is your trouble. Only a physician can determine if your obesity is glandular, and properly prescribe for it. And he can't do it, without thorough tests and examinations. Anything you read will only help you in your understanding of obesity.

Some people believe that if they are fat around the hips and trunk, they have glandular trouble. However, experts point out that heaviness in those parts is common in most cases of obesity—and that it will disappear after diet, even without endocrine treatment. Other fat distribution, thought to be caused by glands, often disappears with diet, too, proving that it was not glandular in origin. As physicians still disagree about glandular obesity, there is no way of describing, definitely, exact glandular cases.

Many physicians believe that the patient with a large trunk and slender wrists and ankles has pituitary obesity. If it is associated with dwarfism, it is known as the Burnier type of obesity. Another type of pituitary obesity is the so-called Cushing's disease, or basophilic adenoma of the pituitary gland. In these patients the obesity is prominent in the girdle region of the body, and develops rapidly. Obesity is confined to the face, neck, thorax and abdomen. The face is round and florid, the breasts large, the abdomen protuberant. This disease is quite rare.

Most of the fat girls in side shows have glandular obesity of the pituitary type. Not always—some of them are just fat from eating more food than their bodies can take care of· But the pituitary abnormal person usually evidences this type of overweight, though even this fat may be hypothalamic and not pituitary. These people have small facial features and small hands and feet. Their fat is found principally in the breasts, abdomen, buttocks, thighs and upper arms. In other words, they have the so-called "girdle" and "apron" of fat. In basal metabolism tests, the metabolism may be below normal level, and the sugar tolerance high. There are often disturbances in salt and water metabolism, too.

The thyroid type of obesity is far more common—though it, too, is rarer than people think. And seldom are there pure thyroid types; often the other glands are involved, too. But don't think that you need thyroid, because you're overweight. Thousands of people have dosed themselves with thyroid extracts when they had no thyroid disturbances at all.

In thyroid obesity—hypothyroid obesity, as it is called —fat is increased to some extent, but there is also a fluid present. This form of overweight is called myxedema. It is determined by a basal metabolism test. This is a simple test, in which the patient fasts all night and the next morning, and then is given pure oxygen to breath, while indications are made on a chart of the amount of oxygen that is breathed. If the basal metabolism is extremely low, the physician believes that the patient has a hypothyroid condition—and if the patient is overweight, he usually prescribes thyroid, in the proper amount, with other medication and diet. Some doctors do not believe that this is a true test for a thyroid deficiency, but it is generally accepted. People with subthyroid function have, usually, a dry skin, coarse, dry hair, lack of perspiration, a slow heart beat and constipation. Obesity in hypothyroidism is usually pretty well distributed all over the body, but there may be quite a bit of fat in the lower part of the neck, the upper part of the back, on the breasts, upper thighs, ankles and legs.

Another form of obesity, though extremely rare, is that attributed to gonadal deficiency. These patients are extremely nervous and emotionally unstable. In women, the fat usually occurs on the buttocks and thighs, and sometimes appears after the menopause. In men, the mammary development is marked, and the patient shows girdle and hip fat, and sometimes female hair distribution. Laboratory tests show a low-normal or decreased sugar tolerance and a decrease in sex hormones. Luckily, this form of obesity is the easiest that a physician has to contend with. The right medication and the patient is on the way to normal weight. Diet, as with all other forms of weight correction, is necessary.

Very occasionally, fat may be caused by a tumor on

one of the glands. Only a physician can determine this, of course. And luckily, this is most rare.

It is practically certain that yours is not a glandular case. But you never know! Only a thorough physical examination will determine this. And certainly, if your case is glandular, you will be helped by medication, together with the diet that is best for you. Even if I were a doctor, which I'm not, I couldn't prescribe for you unless I saw you. Anyone who prescribes, sight unseen, for a person suffering from any disease, should be severely dealt with by the authorities. Even an experienced doctor couldn't prescribe for a patient he hadn't examined.

Never take any medicine for reduction—or for anything else—that is not given to you by a reputable doctor! Thousands of people have ruined their health by taking so-called reduction pills, full of unnecessary laxatives, so-called vitamins (that were usually low in vitamin value), thyroid (when the patient's condition did not call for thyroid), or one of the dangerous drugs that could cause real trouble.

Obesity is a disease. I'm trying to show you the causes of it. You certainly cannot cure it by unauthorized dosages of any medical preparation.

I've known people who were helped by a doctor's prescription to give some of the medicine to a neighbor, in a most mistaken idea of friendliness. I've even known ignorant people to say, "Here, wear my glasses. They may help your eyes," when the prescription for the glasses was carefully written for a particular individual, and could hurt the sight of another person! Nothing to do with obesity? Certainly not. But the person who mistakenly lends his specially ground lenses to another person, and advises medicine for colds or headaches, may well pass along an obesity "cure." Take no medication of any kind for obesity unless a physician prescribes it especially for you.

There are those who do not believe in doctors. Certain religious sects do not believe in consulting physicians. I know an important dietitian who believes that Bernard Shaw died, not because he was ninety-four years old, but because doctors gave him penicillin and other drugs—which brought about uremic poisoning and death. Another dietitian believes that Al Jolson died because of the drugs given him, before he went to Korea, to keep him free from disease while there. These people are sincere. So are thousands more who have similar beliefs. I believe in the miracles of the "miracle" drugs. But I don't believe that anyone should take them without professional prescription, nor that they are for everyone.

If you want to lose weight, and be healthy and strong, my advice to you is, first, to study yourself; second, to go to a good physician for a thorough examination; and third, to do what he tells you to do.

Certainly, you can do nothing about glandular treatment without a physician's help. You may find that in the glands lies the secret of your obesity. It isn't likely—but it's possible. If you have a glandular deficiency, you'll be helped immensely. If not, you'll know the truth about yourself, physically, and will be able to take the necessary steps toward reaching normal weight.

CHAPTER 6

Salt of the earth

AT ONE TIME, you couldn't give a person a higher compliment than saying, "He's the salt of the earth." Lately, salt has lost its savor—and doesn't rank so well. In fact, a lot of experts believe that too much salt is one cause of obesity. A salt-restricted diet has proved successful in many cases of obesity. As with all other reduction diets, it must be taken with a pinch of salt—for the diet calls for far more than salt restriction.

The salt which is said to make fat is, of course, good old sodium chloride. It is found in ocean water and in beds formed by the drying up of ancient bodies of water.

Salt has been important as a seasoning and a preserving agent since prehistoric times. It was used as an altar offering by the ancient Greeks, the Romans and the Hebrews. It was used as an important medium of exchange in commercial ventures across the Mediterranean and the Adriatic seas. It has been subjected to taxation in Oriental countries. It served as money in Ethiopia and Tibet. It caused wars, made peace. The word "salary" comes from the salt allowance made to Roman soldiers. Wild animals go where "salt licks" can be found. It is a universal constituent in diet.

Today, we're told that salt makes fat! Some of the newest and best diets call for salt restriction. They do not call for doing without salt entirely. Weakness may result, if no salt is eaten. Uremia has resulted because of salt depletion. But many successful reduction programs call for a lessening of sodium chloride intake.

Practically all living matter contains salt. We need salt to be healthy. The body fluid of man contains 0.85% salt. This balance is maintained in the blood of all healthy individuals. Any change causes real trouble. Too much salt, the experts say, may cause high blood pressure. And while it does not make fat in itself, it causes water retention—which, the experts tell us, is just as bad. It seems that a change in sodium chloride balance means a change in water balance. The tissues become water-logged. Fluid gathers, and organs are swollen, their natural functions interfered with. The healthy individual can excrete about 10 grams of sodium chloride every twenty-four hours. But if the physiological mechanisms are unbalanced, salt often tends to accumulate, to hold water in the tissue spaces.

In 1922, Dr. Frederick M. Allen found the use of a diet low in sodium chloride excellent for high blood pressure. Since that time, low sodium chloride diets have been found successful in the treatment of many other diseases, and some forms of obesity have yielded to this treatment. Dr. Walter Kempner of Duke University has had great success with his rice diet for high blood pressure—and this, too, has proved helpful in some obesity cases.

This is why Dr. Emil G. Conason approves of the low-salt diet not only for high blood pressure but for weight reduction. He says, "A portion of the weight of the obese person consists of water, bound to sodium in his tissues. This water may be liberated and excreted during the maintenance of the low-sodium diet. In addition, the low-sodium diet tends to decrease the hydrochloric acid production in the stomach, thereby decreasing hunger. Low-sodium diets for reducing will be found of inestimable help in the program of weight reduction." Dr. Conason and Ella Metz, a dietitian, are the authors of *The Salt-Free Diet Cook Book,* published by Lear, and valuable to anyone who wishes to go on a salt-free diet.

I know dozens of women who have reduced their weight by the low-salt method. Like all other diets, it is a method to be considered only if approved by your own physician. Water retention is certainly often a serious cause of overweight.

The usual low-sodium diet calls for liquid restriction, also. The regulation reduction diet is followed, omitting practically all salt. Some salt will be in food, of course, especially if you eat in restaurants. But no extra salt must be added. Besides this, no liquids must be taken at meals. No liquids at all! Between meals, liquids may be taken, the amount depending on your own condition and your own doctor.

Vivian Blaine, the beautiful young actress, whose figure is exceptionally slender and attractive, told me that her successful weight reduction is the result of

liquid restriction. She weighed 150 pounds and was told
she was too fat for the stage or Hollywood. She dieted
down to 130 pounds, then couldn't lose another ounce,
    "The studio thought I was cheating," she told me.
"I wasn't at all. I ate what I was told. But I drank a
lot of water and juices, with meals, too. Then another
doctor put me on a water-restricted diet. I drink only
four glasses of water a day—and not with meals. My
weight is 115 pounds—which is just right for me. Of
course, I'm still careful of my diet—and of the amount
of liquids I consume."

Four women prominent in public life have recently
lost twenty pounds each by giving up salt—and water—
at their meals.

If you are on a low-salt diet and can't enjoy your
food without the flavor that salt gives it, I can recommend a number of substitutes. There are dozens of
substitutes on sale at the health shops. The one I like
best is "Diasal," manufactured by E. Fourgera, and
consisting of potassium chloride and glutamic acid.
"Fortissimo Brand Seasoning," made by Isrin-Oliver,
"Gustamate," made by the Arlington Chemical Company, and "Co-Salt," made by Cassimir Funk Laboratories, are all good, too. Not nearly as good as real
salt—sodium chloride—but very satisfactory for seasoning, when sodium is not indicated.

Of course you've heard of Dr. Kempner's famous
rice diet. Originally introduced for high blood pressure,
it has found great success among many people who are
overweight. My objection to it is that it is monotonous.

My idea of a good diet is one that can be kept up indefinitely as a way of living. The Kempner diet is not that by any means. But because it is salt-free and has been discussed a great deal, I think it has a place here. The diet consists only of rice, fruit, fruit juice and sugar or honey. No water! No salt! The rice is boiled. It may be white, polished, brown or wild. The fruit may be raw, stewed, canned, dried, frozen or preserved. Nuts, dates and avocados are forbidden. The sugar may be white, brown or honey—but no commercial syrups may be used. Vegetable juices are *not* included. Liquids are limited to a pint and a half or two pints of fruit juices, canned or fresh. A vitamin and iron supplement is recommended. Dr. Kempner has found that the diet results in a significant reduction in the size of greatly enlarged hearts and that water-logging, due to kidney disease, is eliminated.

A short stay on the rice diet may be of benefit to the overweight person who has water retention and high blood pressure. It should be taken only on the advice and under the supervision of a competent physician. While it was never planned just for the obese, it may be just what some fat people need. I don't recommend it as a "way of life," or a permanent weight-reducer.

This isn't at all what I have in mind for you. It's a sort of stop by the wayside, a trip up a side street. Because the low-sodium and water-restricted diet is being discussed so much today, I felt that we should discuss it, too. Now we're on our way to thinking ourselves thin . . . .

CHAPTER 7

This may
be the answer

YOU'RE FAT BECAUSE YOU OVEREAT. That is, you eat too much for your particular body, your particular mechanism. It might not be too much for some people. But it's too much for you. And it undoubtedly is not your glands. And it probably isn't your salt-and-water retention. It's food! Food makes fat! Heard that before? You'll hear it again. If you're writing down what you eat each night, you ought to have about a week's record, now. I hope so, at any rate. Before too long a time, you'll be able to prove to yourself exactly how much too much you're eating—and what foods are fattening for you. And then you'll know what to eat, and what not to eat.

Now, you've another problem. It's to decide why you overeat. When you've found that out, you've solved one of the greatest problems of obesity. It's quite possible that you've never found out the reason. Nor considered the reason important. Once you've found it out—and faced it—you'll be able to solve your own special obesity problem with no trouble at all. You may even enjoy getting thin! That may sound difficult—impossible—to you, but it isn't. I wish you'd see the people who have changed, practically overnight, because their viewpoints have changed. Literally, they've been able to think themselves thin.

There are many reasons for overeating. I won't be able to take up all of them, but I'll touch on the most important reasons. I think—and hope—I'll find the one that is pertinent to your particular case. If I don't, you may be able to discover it by yourself. But if I do find 'out why you are fat, please accept it. Don't shy away from it and say, "Oh, that doesn't suit me at all!" The sooner you find the facts that fit you, the sooner you'll be able to think yourself thin. Face it! There's a reason why you overeat. Once you discover the reason, it will be far easier for you to stop pigging. It's a fault, like biting your fingernails, only far harder on your figure and your health. It will be difficult for you to break the habit of overeating. But once you face the reasons, the habit will be far more easily conquered. Dieting without knowing the reasons back of it is too much like trying to wear a suit or a dress that is made for someone else. It may be a fine garment, but if it isn't made for you, what good is it for you? You might have to force yourself to accept it because you haven't anything better. But now, you'll have something better. Your own personal reason for being your better self.

You needn't tell anyone of your findings. If you like, it can be your own secret. I can't possibly know! No one else will know—unless you tell. Tell—if you like.

That's up to you. But accept it for yourself. So, here we go!

The reason you're fat may be something that happened before you were born! So you can't be blamed for it. But, knowing the reason, you can correct the fault.

First, you may have inherited a tendency for fat. Not that you inherited the fat itself. But if all of your family was fat, especially your mother's family, you may well have inherited a fat tendency. Another thing—if your mother and your mother's family was fat, that usually means that they "lived well." The table was always set with the delicacies of the season, and there was an abundance of everything. So you ate a great deal when you were young—were encouraged to eat. And two things happened. You gained a liking for good food, and you gained the habit of eating a great deal.

Families that "set a good table" always encourage the children to eat a great deal. To those families, healthy children are fat children.

But let's go back again to the days before you were born. You may well have come from a fat-prone family. Perhaps your mother was fat before you were born. So, even before you were born, you received too much nourishment—gained a pre-natal conception of food. That means you've always been fat. Impossible to get thin now? Not at all. You've only been fat too long—and you can get thin, if you really want to.

On the other hand, you may have been a thin baby. Perhaps, while your mother carried you, you were too thin.

So, even before you were born, you were hungry. Coming into the world a thin, hungry baby, you craved food—and have been craving it ever since. That, too, is understood by obesity experts. Your desire for food has always been with you. You can get rid of that, too, just by facing facts. You aren't hungry, now. There's no need for you to keep on overeating!

The family that lived in luxury set a luxury pattern that is extremely hard to break. The fat adult who lived with rich foods as a child has the subconscious idea that he is "stepping down" from his position of luxury if he eats plainer food. If he can convince himself that this is not so, it will be easy enough for him to accept the foods that must be good for him, now.

I weighed less than five pounds when I was born. I was a scrawny, small baby, born in a Southern family that loved luxury. I was an only child. Immediately, the whole family—parents, grandparents and servants— then, in the South, a house full of servants didn't mean unusual opulence—had one object in mind—to fatten the baby. I grew fat. By the time I was a year old, I was round and chubby. And I stayed that way. Considering the family meals, it's a wonder any of us was able to waddle around, not alone walk. Curiously enough, my father stayed quite slender; my mother and grandmother were only a bit overweight—with nice, old-fashioned, high-stomached figures. I was the fat one! Because of my pre-birth hunger? Probably. But most likely because I had a large appetite—and ate huge meals. The only wonder was that I wasn't fat enough for a side show. I'm less than 5 feet 2 inches, and when I went away to college I weighed nearly 150 pounds—a large, fat girl. I don't know, now, how I managed to have fun. But I did. I lost a little weight at college. The meals weren't so good and the gymnasium was. But I wasn't thin. It wasn't until a few years ago that I said to myself, "Face it!" and decided that the time had come to reduce. Then I got my weight under some sort of control. Now I weigh around no pounds—and I'm never going to weigh much more, if I can help it.

Those Arkansas meals! I can enjoy them now, in retrospect. Certainly, I can't eat meals like that, now. Nor can anyone I know.

Our breakfasts, in those days, consisted of a bit of fruit—no one cared a lot for fruit at meals, though. Fruit was something to nibble between meals. There was always a bowl of fruit on the sideboard, and a couple of big Arkansas apples, or two or three Arkansas peaches, were just an in-between-meals snack, not to be counted at all. The grown-ups had several cups of coffee each. My grandmother didn't take sugar in her coffee, I remember. Just cream. But she liked two or three cups of it. The rest of the family took cream and sugar. I was given an imitation of coffee, consisting of rich Arkansas milk—so yellow with cream it resembled the "light" cream of today—spiked a bit with coffee to give it color, and with cream and sugar to give it flavor. After the fruit, there were always ham and eggs or bacon and eggs—the eggs usually made into an omelet or scrambled with cream. This was served with hot

bread, usually biscuits or muffins, which were accompanied by country butter—"take two and butter 'em while
they're hot"—and, of course, home-made preserves,
usually two kinds. Hot breads were served three times
a day in Arkansas. Once in a while, we could have very
fresh, very warm "light bread"—but if you had light
bread too often, you were put down as "Poor White,"
or worse, "Northerners," who, of course, couldn't
know any better. That, with a bit of cottage cheese,
rich with cream, was all we ever had for breakfast,
week-days. On Sundays, of course, breakfasts were a
bit heavier. Then, besides the other things, there were
always pancakes or waffles—usually waffles—to be
smothered in butter, so that every little indentation was
"full up," and then covered all over with maple syrup,
which ran off the waffle onto the plate. These were always accompanied by little sausages in Winter—crisp
and brown—and by curls of bacon, when the weather
grew too warm for sausages.

The mid-day meal—it was called dinner when I was
very young, but got changed to "lunch" as I grew
older, just as supper at night became, more stylishly,
"dinner"—was a simple one, as my father had to go
back to the store—he had a wholesale store that sup-
plied the little country stores in the nearby towns—and
I had to go back to school or to play. For lunch there
was home-made soup. Sultan, my Saint Bernard, got
the bone, which would readily pass for a very good pot
roast today. The soup was a thick one, and usually contained home-made noodles, and bits of meat, rice or

vegetables. Then came the meat course: pot roast or chicken—not very expensive in Arkansas—or baked ham or tongue, in a sauce rich with gingersnaps and raisins, or roast lamb, or perhaps a stuffed shoulder of lamb, or roast beef. With this went hominy or black-eyed peas or potatoes, usually baked with the meat, if possible, or mashed to a fluff with butter and cream, or a couple of vegetables drenched with butter, hot bread*—usually cornbread in squares—to be broken open and slathered with butter. Salads were as unimportant as the fruit at breakfast, but, when there was salad, it was rich with dressing and chopped eggs—as was the spinach. Dessert was pie, more than likely, with a cheese accompaniment, or a hot pudding, a custard or home-made cake with a thick sauce.

After school, of course, I had to have something to eat. Wasn't I a growing girl? Nothing elaborate, of course. Just a pocketful of cookies, covered with chopped nuts, if I was at home. Or an ice cream soda—or two—if I was out with "the crowd." Supper was early. And even when it became "dinner," it wasn't any more elaborate than the mid-day meal. Just a roast and vegetables and potatoes or hominy and dessert. Hot bread, of course. And home-made preserves. The family especially liked fried chicken or dishes with Creole sauce. Sweet potatoes, covered with brown sugar and marshmallows and baked until the top was brown, were a frequent meat accompaniment. The sweet pickles were home-made, too. And so was the ice cream—usually a sort of frozen custard, rich with cream and eggs.

Before I went to bed at night, I got nothing but a few pieces of chocolate—milk chocolate in colored foil wrappings that my mother bought especially for me, and a glass of milk accompanied by a piece of nearly plain cake or a few cookies. Of course, when there was company, I was allowed to taste of the late-supper delicacies—a bit of pink baked ham, a nibble of imported cheese, a stuffed "devilled" egg, a few beaten biscuits or cold fried chicken, finished off with a dish of ice cream or sherbet or fruit cake.

So you can see why, even now, it's hard for me to stay on the diet I try to follow, and why I've invented special dishes in an effort to recapture some of the forbidden flavors of my youth. But I do diet, which îs better for my figure and, I believe, for my health, than if I stuck with the Arkansas menus of my youth.

Your own problem is undoubtedly a much different one. But I thought you might like to know what I've been up against.

Instead of the luxuries of childhood, the fat person, today, may have had an entirely different upbringing. He may have been too poor. The fare may have been too meager. So he dreamed of the time he could eat all he wanted of rich and, at that time, unattainable food. Food represents to him luxury and, in a way, success. They tell me that when you see a fat man in a restaurant surrounded by young and attractive people—younger and more attractive than he is—and when he is obviously the host, that he is compensating for past poverty and present fat by giving lavishly. Showing that, as host, he is important, fits in. If he'd diet he'd feel better—and probably live longer and be just as popular. But his very weight—his unnecessary fat— represents, to him, his material success. To those who understand him, it sometimes represents the poverty of his youth—in a way, the fulfillment of his dreams. When he faces things—faces himself—he'll pay more attention to his inner needs, and less attention to attracting others. He'll diet, get a chance to look and feel well, and find that he's more successful, and has more friends than ever before.

You may be fat because you're afraid. Maybe you were afraid when you were young, and your present fear is just a hangover. Or you may be afraid, now— and Heaven knows there's enough to be afraid of. You eat because of fear. To convince yourself that you have enough of everything, that the world is a stable, firm place, that everything is all right, that creature comforts are right here for you—and always will be. The way things are now, we can't be sure of anything, as we realize. But gobbling up a lot of unnecessary calories in order to convince yourself that you're safe and comfortable isn't going to help things at all. Do something useful, instead, and you'll feel and look better. Remember, the food you eat today isn't going to help a bit tomorrow! Don't be a squirrel and garner food and possessions. Eat your needs, today; do the best you can—and let tomorrow take care of itself. The extra food you eat today isn't really doing a bit of good toward helping your fear—of today—of tomorrow—of anything.

The conceited person is sometimes too fat. He says to himself, "I'm absolutely right about everything. Eating is right—for me. I'm attractive enough looking, fat or thin." Of course he isn't! The fat woman who thinks she's perfection and that her fat is attractive ought to face herself the way she really is. If she'll do that, her very conceit will cause her to do something definite—and get thin in no time at all.

There are a lot more types of people who could think themselves thin, once they put their minds to it. Which one are you?

CHAPTER 8

Face it-

you're fat!

THERE ARE SO MANY PEOPLE in the world who arc thinking themselves fat when they could think themselves thin, instead, once they see the facts—and themselves—in the right light.

There's the person with the Inferiority Complex— that good old Inferiority Complex that the psychiatrists and psychoanalysts have been talking about! You'd never think that it would have anything to do with getting fat. But it has a lot to do with it. Thousands of people—maybe hundreds of thousands—eat too much, to compensate for an Inferiority Complex. Could, by any chance, one of these be you?

One of the most prevalent examples of obesity of this type is the unpopular fat girl who doesn't go places or do things like other girls. Instead, she stays home— and eats. Food is her solace, her excuse, her companion.

This girl isn't unpopular because she's fat—though that is what she likes to tell herself. She's fat because she's unpopular. She's unpopular because she's afraid, and has an Inferiority Complex. Let's start at the beginning. Perhaps the girl is already slightly fat. Perhaps she comes of a fat-prone family. Or maybe she isn't fat at all, but for some reason, she doesn't fit in. Or thinks she doesn't. People, she believes, do not like her. Young men do not ask for dates—aren't attracted to her when they meet her. Instead of learning how to attract men by the good old rules of getting better looking and learning to talk—and learning to flatter men and appear provocative—she turns to food.

She doesn't have to be popular to eat the things she likes. She really doesn't like men, she tells herself. She much prefers chocolate creams and whipped cream desserts. They won't turn against her! Oh, won't they, just! If she'd only see it!

As she becomes fat—which she will, sure as Fate, if she turns to rich foods for solace—she has a fine alibi for her unpopularity. She is unpopular because she is fat! So she hides behind her fat. Her extra weight is her screen, her comfort, her excuse for everything.

This girl can get thin—can lose her disguise of awkward and ugly fat very easily—once she has faced the facts, and herself. All she has to do is to get her medical checkup, and go on a strict "think yourself thin" regime. She has to turn from herself—from food, from goodies—to the world. She has to learn how to interest herself in people. One of the beauty schools is an ideal starter for her. Here she'll meet other girls, see people who have almost her own problem. A good gymnasium would be a fine help, if the beauty school isn't convenient. Or she can just exercise at home, and take long walks—and force herself into outside activities.

She can do the things that popular girls do—and learn the little tricks that attract men. And say, "You're wonderful!" to the men she meets, instead of reaching for that extra piece of pastry.

Recently, I took a trip with a group of girls. I won't say which group—I've taken several trips. Almost immediately there were two cliques. They divided themselves without any help from anyone. There were the girls who spent most of their time at the table. At breakfast, they took twice as much time as the other girls. At luncheon, food was important. They talked about the food, ate eagerly. At cocktail time, they drank and ate avidly. At dinner—usually a buffet dinner—they chose their food carefully, went back for second helpings, ate as much as they could. And they usually ate before they went to bed. They didn't get much out of the trip except a few extra pounds. Most of their conversation was about how much they were eating, and the quality and quantity of the food. The other girls were too busy to bother much about food. Oh, they ate—and ate well I Food was important to them—but important as just one of the treats of the trip. They were too busy seeing things and doing things to pay too much attention to what they were eating. At meal time, they concentrated on food. But when meals were over, they were off to see things, to have fun. They ran around at a great rate, saw all the sights, met new people, made new friends, came home bubbling over with new ideas, new memories, a real and lasting impression of other ways of life—something they could use always. The eaters came home with only the memory of food—food they'd have been better off without. I won't say that all of the eaters had an Inferiority Complex. Some of their eating habits may have been acquired in other ways. But they ate their way around, and lost out on everything else. Even if you stay home you can have a better time if you turn to other things for pleasure— and accept the pleasures of the table as just one of the good things in life, while you're hunting for, and enjoying, the others.

Men have the same complex, though it may hit them a bit differently. The fat man with an Inferiority Complex likes to think that he is an introvert and just can't be bothered with people, when, actually, he longs for popularity. He eats instead of getting out and meeting people. Some of the eaters, among men, don't get fat. They all get unpopular—and a lot of them do gain unwanted weight, too. If they followed the same rules, they'd lose, too. And be far happier, fit into their world better, make a place for themselves where they'd be important and popular for themselves—not just take up space—and maybe too much space.

These aren't the only people who are fat because they eat too much. Certainly not! There are the emotional wrecks. They don't look like wrecks. They just look round, and even unemotional. You wouldn't think, looking at them devouring their food, that they are seething inside, dissatisfied, worried, miserable, frightened. Things go wrong—and they eat. They can't get the things they want in the world, so they turn to food.

They can't get the job they'd like to have, so they take out their emotions on puddings and apple pies. It's so comforting to eat a box of butter creams when things go wrong! To turn to salted nuts when the telephone doesn't ring. To go to an expensive restaurant for an elegant and fattening meal when some other wish has been denied. They're afraid for the state of the world —so they eat too much!

It seems so simple—for an outsider! If the worrier could only turn to some other help, have another out-let! And he can, once he sees that he is eating himself into more worry, into illness—perhaps shortening his life. All the worrier has to do is to face facts and see that food isn't enough—isn't the answer at all. There are so many things the worrier can do, instead. Useful things. Pleasant things. He can mix with people, learn a new avocation.

I know of remarkable cures of worriers who were eaters. One was a girl who had had an unfortunate love affair. She was miserable, and felt that everyone knew she'd been left practically at the altar. As a matter of fact, not too many people knew—and practically no one cared. The girl worried herself into becoming a wreck—a fat wreck. She ate constantly; food was her only comfort. She grew fat and ugly—and told herself that the reason no one paid any attention to her was because she was fat. But she kept on worrying and suffering.

Luckily, that wasn't the end—for her. She became ill, and was fortunate enough to consult a physician who was more interested in her mental condition than in her slight physical ailment. He talked to her—got some of the facts. She was willing to try his remedy. She went on a diet. Started to exercise. Turned to a completely new way of living. In six months she'd thought herself thin. In eight months she had become popular, was having a fine time. Now she's happily married—and still slender. She thinks a miracle happened to her. She just "came to herself," faced facts and thought herself thin.

Many other people have grown fat and unattractive and unhappy because of unfortunate love affairs. These people with broken hearts may be either male or female. I've known a number of men who have exchanged broken hearts for too-fat bodies. Usually, though, it's the woman who mopes around and gets too fat because of an unsatisfactory love affair.

A well-known actress, who is usually in an emotional upheaval, tells me that she gets fat only when she's unhappy.

"When I'm happy, I don't think about eating," she told me. "But I fall in love, and things don't go so well. So I stay at home and eat. I run to the refrigerator—when the telephone doesn't ring. I eat chocolates when I stay home in the evening and mope. I grow fat, and lose my figure and have an awful time of it"

Luckily, for her, she has to make a living—has to take hold of herself, face facts, and her lost figure. So she diets down to correct weight—and gets a job, and finds new happiness.

Unrequited love is not helped by food. Food isn't even a good substitute for affection. I know it is easy for me to say, "Get interested in someone else—in something else!" But, actually, that is the only answer. Turning to food will mean only that you'll lose your figure, and perhaps your health, and be farther away from affection and happiness than ever. Even the most popular and desirable individuals have unfortunate affairs of the heart, and think that life isn't worth living. It's better to have emotional upheavals than never to have emotions at all. But don't turn to food for solace! Excess food is not your friend and comforter. Turn to people, to new interests. Getting fat will just add another problem—it won't solve a thing. Face it—and get a new figure and a new heart interest.

Then there is the nibbler. He—or she—is a worrier, too. Worries about little things. And nibbles all day long. If it's a man, he always has candy or nuts in his pocket, or rushes into a lunch room half a dozen times a day for a cup of coffee and a sweet roll or a piece of cake. Or he drinks too much, and eats while he drinks. The woman nibbler eats all day long, at home or in business. I know women nibblers who spend most of the day trailing to the kitchen and back again. They don't eat much at a time. Certainly not I Just a cookie or bunch of grapes or an apple or a piece of bread covered with cream cheese and preserves. Or they nibble at the candy or nuts that they keep on the living room coffee table. The nibbler is nervous and takes out his nerves on food. Someone said that the proof of an iron will is to be able to eat exactly three salted nuts. The nibbler might try that, for a starter.

Like the others who must think themselves thin, the nibbler can cure himself. Once he faces facts. At the table, he probably doesn't eat more than anyone else. Not much more 1 His secret nibbles alone would supply enough calories to keep him well-fed. Once he faces facts, he can begin to lead a normal and healthy life, and become slender and well-balanced. I know a former nibbler who has turned into a well-balanced, happy—and slender—person. He still eats five meals a day. Insists on tea, and a bite before he goes to bed. But his meals are well-balanced. He's learned what to eat. And he's given up most of his nibbling. No longer do his pockets bulge with chocolate bars and salted nuts.

Another person who eats too much is the young bride. There are an awful lot of cases of young-matron obesity. The young bride, whether she is at home or still holding her job, suddenly lets down. She's accomplished one of her aims. She's got her man! Overcome by her own cleverness in landing him, her own satisfaction in getting married, she stops trying. She's got what she wanted, hasn't she? Why keep on struggling? She doesn't realize that getting a man is only one step. Holding him is the next step—but she hasn't thought that far ahead.

The young bride at home has the hardest time of it.

That new kitchen! The chance to eat anything she wants to eat at any time! She cooks—and tastes. And, during the day, finishes up the left-overs. If she's at home, she usually doesn't have enough to do. Eating takes up her extra time. It's fun, eating anything she wants to eat at any time. She's got her man. She might as well enjoy herself.

The young bride, at home or in business, who loses her figure, is going to find that she has eaten herself out of happiness. The time for her to get hold of herself is before she has gained ten pounds. If she's already gained them, the time is now! She can think herself thin easily enough, once she realizes what has happened to her.

The young matron who has started to raise a family is in an even more dangerous position in regard to her fat and her future. While she is pregnant, it is so easy for her to gain weight. Although her doctor tells her how much she may gain with safety, she frequently gains too much. Even if she doesn't, and if she's careful about her weight, following all the rules, after the baby comes she is apt to let down. She can't get out as much. And she's pretty satisfied with herself and her family. Chocolate cake and rich cream desserts take the place of more active pleasures. She can't go out and leave the baby. But she can—and does—stay home and gobble rich foods. It's a hard job to hold out, when the kitchen is full of good things to eat and there's not a thing to do but eat them. But even the young mother can face life realistically and see that a slim young matron is going to have a better future than a fat girl, who is bound to move—and think—a bit slower than she should. To keep her husband interested, to be a good mother and wife and citizen, she should force herself to have enough interests so that the joys of eating become relatively unimportant. She has so much to be thankful for. She doesn't need superfluous food as one of her blessings.

The middle-aged man or woman who "lets down," and lets food take the place of other interests, is well known to all of us, even if we've never thought of him —or her—in that way. They've found their places in the world. They become smug, self-satisfied, dull—and fat.

These middle-aged, fat dullards can be divided into two classes by that good old divider—money. The poorer middle-aged men or women decide there is nothing more for them—so they settle back, dissatisfied, and perhaps frightened about practically everything but the pleasures of the table. Or they aren't dissatisfied, but just settle down. They have the radio and television. They aren't interested in other people, and the world holds little for them. The food which is easiest to get—and which they can best afford—is fattening food: potatoes, rice, bread and jelly. Sometimes beer is added as food. They stop thinking, and grow fat, instead. There is still a chance for these people to get something out of life and enjoy other things besides eating, if they'll start thinking about it.

The middle-aged couples with money who become

too fat have the same problem. Only they have become fat, usually, as their one means of self-expres-
sion. It pleases them to be able to eat in good restaurants, order expensive foods. In a way, it represents
success. Every pound they gain costs them money. It
is their outward expression of inward smugness. Here's
a secret for them: it will cost them just as much to get
thin as it did to grow fat. As they like to spend money,
that should please them. One "society" expert in New
York figures that it costs his richest patients one hundred dollars a pound to reduce—that includes his expensive services and the massage and food that he prescribes. A girl I know, and not a rich girl, either, tells
me it cost her thirty dollars a pound to lose weight,
with medical advice, diet and supervised exercise. It
needn't cost that, of course. But rich folks who love to
spend money can spend it most satisfactorily on losing
weight. They'll enjoy losing it far more if it is costing
them a lot of money. To them, spending is a sign of
power. If they want to lose weight, they can lose weight,
and spend money doing it. And they may even find that
they have new interests and can find other things on
which to spend their money. The size 12 mutation mink
coat can cost just as much as the size 40, you know!
And diamonds cost just as much in settings sized to
fit the smaller wrist, finger or neck. The fat matron
may find, if she loses weight, that she'll actually gain
the sort of popularity she likes to believe she has now.
The fat man-about-town may actually be liked for him-

self, once he stops being smug, pompous, dull and over-weight.

There are dozens of other types of overweights—but I think you get the idea. If you're too fat, try to find out why you eat too much—for you may as well take it for granted that you do. Once you find out why you overeat, you're on the road not only to a better figure but to better health, better adjustment—and a far more interesting and well-balanced life. Isn't it about time that you began to think yourself thin?

Are you writing down, every night, every bite you eat? It's the only way you can start to think yourself thin, according to my method. Before too long, you're going to analyze your own eating habits, to see if you eat too much, or eat the wrong things. You can't do that if you don't have your data. So keep on collecting it. Now you're trying to find out why you eat too much. Once you've found that out, it's going to be simple enough to discover that you do eat too much of the things that aren't right for you.

CHAPTER 9

Body and soul

You MAY BE TOO FAT—and I take it for granted that you are too fat, or why on earth would you be reading this?—just because you like good food; because food is more important to you than looking well, or being well, or giving yourself a chance at a longer life. Food is mighty comforting. A fine escape. A fine refuge, if you're insecure. But perhaps you're beginning to discover, if you haven't discovered it before, that there is a relationship between you and what you eat—between the person you should be and the food you should be getting. Mind and body, stomach and brain, the things you'd like to do, the person you'd like to be, and the foods that go into your mouth are all closely related. So closely related, in fact, that doctors and psychologists and psychiatrists are studying these relationships more and more.

This treating of mind and body as one unit—and just try to separate them—is called the psychosomatic approach. It is the common ground where psychiatry and the different branches of medicine get together. If you're interested—and I hope you are—read *Psychosomatic Medicine* by Dr. Franz Alexander, published by W. W.

Norton. Dr. Alexander goes much more deeply into the subject than I possibly can here. But perhaps I can give you some of the principles of the psychosomatic approach, as worked out by Dr. Alexander and a number of other psychiatrists, which may start you on the right track, and help you with your own particular problem. Dr. Alexander, by the way, is the Director at the Chicago Institute for Psychoanalysis, and Clinical Professor of Psychiatry at the University of Illinois. Dr. Therese Benedek, whom I shall also quote, is a member of the staff at the Chicago Institute for Psychoanalysis. Don't dismiss psychosomatic medicine as nonsense. And don't tell me that your mind and body aren't closely knit together! Nor that obesity doesn't arise from a combination of the two. In fact, you can think yourself thin only because the parts of that complex organization that is you are so closely knit together. While you're alive, you can't separate mind and body—body and soul. After you're dead? There does seem to be a separation there—which rather proves the point. For the present, I'm not carrying this into a future world. All I want to do is to help you know yourself, and conquer yourself—at least the parts of you that are too fat—while you're still around.

I'm sure you are advanced enough mentally to know that your physical condition influences your mental state. And that, too, on the other hand, your mind influences your body. If you are even mildly confused mentally, or even mildly ill, physically, you need expert treatment—from physician and psychiatrist, who should work together. Psychiatry and neurology have been studied together, so, at long last, patients can be treated simultaneously for illnesses that can only yield to this dual treatment.

But you may not be actually ill. You may be well enough so that an understanding of your own symptoms is all you need to enable you to adjust comfortably to living—and get enough happiness and success out of life, with only a necessary mental check-up, to become thoroughly satisfied as a person. And an attractive and slender person at the same time I

So, perhaps you are fat because of this psychosomatic mixture. For example, chronic emotional disturbances— emotional unhappiness that has lasted for years—may cause endocrine disorders. It has been found that cases of toxic goiter have actually started because of emotional troubles. The mind influenced the glands. They, in turn, influenced the body. The persons become physically ill because of mental upsets. But that is only one small phase of this influence of mind over matter. The carbohydrate metabolism—or the metabolism of sugars and starches— has been found to have been so disturbed by emotions that not only did patients become fat, but they actually developed diabetes.

So here is something to think about. Many chronic internal causes of obesity are the continual functional troubles that come from everyday life, as a person struggles to get along. Emotional conflicts—which psychiatrists recognize as the basis of neuroses—are actually also the cause of certain functional and organic disorders. We eat too much because we are afraid, or insecure, or unhappy.

Or because eating has become too important—because we like to eat. And we get fat. But that isn't all. Not nearly all! Fear, frustrated wishes, all of the other emotions, if we suppress them, can actually result in permanent emotional tensions which physically disturb our vegetative organs.

You see, it's a sort of complicated circle. Our social life is complicated. We have many emotions that cannot be expressed freely. So we divert them into inappropriate channels. We're repressed—so we eat too much ! But that isn't all. The actual repression causes physical trouble— perhaps in metabolism or digestion. So we get fat from that, too! A double dose of blubber because we worry! We eat too much because we're not well adjusted. We get into trouble with our metabolism because we are not well adjusted. And the fat piles up ! Only proper thinking can work a cure. Actually a double cure—just as we had double trouble. Once we find the cause and correct that, then we stop eating too much. And we stop worrying too much. When we stop worrying, our metabolism improves. When we stop worrying, we stop eating too much. With improved metabolism and smaller food intake, we become well adjusted—well physically and slender, all at the same time. We prove, simultaneously, that mind and body work together, that fat makes food and that we can think ourselves thin.

This is one cause of obesity. It may not be the cause of your obesity at all. Psychosomatic—as a term—only means the method of approach, both in research and in therapy. And Dr. Alexander points out, "For example, nostalgic longings and the desire to receive help and affection also stimulate gastric activity. They represent certain brain processes, yet they can be described meaningfully only in psychological terms, because receptive longings cannot at this time be identified by biochemical, electrical or any other non-psychological technique. These brain processes are subjectively perceived as emotions and can be conveyed to others by speech. They can be studied psychologically, and, what is more important, they can be studied adequately only by psychological means."

There are innumerable examples to show that people may be ill because of mental distress. One patient suffered from a gastric neurosis connected with chronic hyperacidity. Whenever he saw a motion picture in which a hero was fighting, or was a dangerous, aggressive character, he had acute heartburn. He identified himself with the hero—but retreated from fighting to get security and help. Such desires for security are closely and intimately connected with the wish to be fed, and so produce increased activities in the stomach.

According to Dr. Alexander, the large group of so-called functional disturbances of the gastrointestinal tract belong in this classification. One of the first emotional tensions perceived by a child is hunger, which, when relieved, is followed by a pleasant feeling of satiation. This starts a pattern for relieving unsatisfied needs. So adults, under emotion, frequently eat too much. And this, in turn, may cause carbohydrate metabolism disturbances. And there we are again!

So, say the experts, any emotion may cause an organic

disturbance, and, because we're interested principally in obesity, we can find out, from the experiments that these experts have made, that frequently actual causes of obesity may be deeper than appear on the surface. We eat too much. And if we eat too much because we are disturbed, then the actual disturbance may cause a metaballistic disturbance. Repressed hostility, erotic impulses, frustration, inferiority or guilt feelings may actually cause vegetative disturbances in themselves—besides causing us to eat too much. Psychologically, our experiences vary. We may wish to be catered to, petted, praised, encouraged or loved. And these very desires, natural though they are, if they are repressed may cause actual physical trouble—a disturbed metabolism. So, when we eat—and under the circumstances we're apt to eat too much—our food does "turn into fat" far too easily.

There is a very real relation between emotion and certain vegetative innervations. They are not vague or mysterious at all, but very definite. For example, our present sophisticated idea of living puts great stress on personal accomplishment—therefore, there are many peptic ulcer patients among the active, ambitious go-getters. So many of us are emotionally unsure, unhappy, dissatisfied. And so many of us are overweight, too. If we become emotionally balanced and satisfied, a lot of the vegetative troubles would take care of themselves.

Considering gastrointestinal disturbances, it may interest you to know that experts have found that in one hundred cases of persecutory delusion, seventy-two per cent suffered from constipation. Persons suffering from depression are also apt to be constipated. They feel rejected and do not expect to receive anything from others. Hence their tendency to hold on to their possessions in the most primitive form of possession, the intestinal content.

Chronic constipation is often considered a trivial symptom, though it is not trivial at all. It is frequently present in obesity. In most cases, diet, laxatives, enemas and massage are used for all practical purposes. But constipation, especially in obesity, may be the manifestation of a deep emotional disturbance. Uncovering the unconscious conflicts often achieves excellent results—both for the constipation and the obesity. Many people who have used laxatives for years have been able to go without them as soon as they learn, by psychotherapy, what is wrong with them.

Constipation is only one—and often not even the most significant—manifestation of an emotional disturbance. A reorientation of the total personality will often cure constipation and will often cure the causes of obesity at the same time.

One of the most important factors in the genesis of the clinical syndrome of diabetes is obesity. However, obesity, in itself, cannot actually be considered a cause of diabetes, as only about five per cent of obese persons develop diabetes. But there is ample evidence to show that obesity does actually produce an increased demand for insulin. When the pancreatic capacity is adequate, according to Dr. Alexander, the increased demand for insulin is compensated for. "In these obese patients," says

Dr. Alexander, "in whom the rate of insulin destruction or utilization is excessive and beyond the use of the regulatory mechanism, a relative insulin insufficiency, and eventually, diabetes, will develop. Overeating is usually the result of some disturbance in the emotional development of the individual. Consequently, psychological factors are etiologically important in those patients who develop diabetes mellitus in consequence of overeating."

Of course, diabetes may develop from many other causes. And obesity, emotionally, is dangerous in itself, as well as because of what it may bring about.

Every organic symptom has an emotional significance of which the ego takes advantage for the relief of emotional annoyance. Being fat takes care of a lot of emotional troubles. The fat person hides behind his fat. He blames his superfluous weight for a lot of things. So, once he becomes normal in weight, he has a new problem. He has new responsibilities. He has nothing to hide behind! He wants to be slender—but often he is too neurotic to accept slenderness.

A person may become slender, physically, after much dieting and trouble, and still remain ill, psychologically. That is why so many people diet and get thin—and then get even fatter, once their dieting days are over. To become slender and remain slender, the obese person—the ill person—must be well psychologically as well as physically.

The psychosomatic approach to obesity means that the fat person cannot divide his problem into physical and mental states. He must be treated by teamwork—co-operation that treats both mental and physical ailments.

The fat person with a psychosomatic basis for obesity will get thin, and stay thin, when he knows himself. When he is able to express his pent-up hostile emotions, or gets over his reasons for feeling guilty. Then he can get over wanting to be fat—a subconscious wanting. He will no longer want to hide behind fat, but will want to be himself, and take his place in the world as a well-balanced and efficient person.

The well-adjusted person who was once fat will still enjoy eating. But eating will no longer be one of the most important things in the world. Eating will take its rightful place, for nourishment, for enjoyment. But the well person will no longer eat for escape—either because the eating for pleasure is a substitute for other things, or because the actual fat is necessary as a screen. And the well-adjusted person will stay slender, both because his metabolism will be more nearly normal, and because food will take its necessary place in his life.

How to become well-adjusted? That may be a job for a psychiatrist, or a trained psychologist. Or a person may be able to analyze himself, once his physical adjustment has been made. But there must be two adjustments —one mental and the other physical. For many people, only through a psychosomatic approach can a real success in reduction be secured.

Here is an experiment you may want to try. It is not one of the "necessary" things for thinking yourself thin, such as writing down, each morning, the amount you weigh, and, each night, the things you've eaten. But it has often helped people who are not too emotionally disturbed, and who are able to help themselves.

Buy a small note book. Those note books, again 1 Get a strong rubber band and a pen or pencil. Those are all you'll need. Each morning, as soon as you wake up, write down, for five minutes, all of your thoughts. Try to remember your dreams, if you can. No matter how confused or vague they are, write them down! If you can't remember your dreams, write down all of the stray thoughts that run through your mind. Write down every thought, no matter how foolish or vague! Don't try to be literary! Just write! For exactly five minutes. Then turn the page of the note book—and put a rubber band around the pages you've written.

The next morning, write again for five minutes. Do not read what you've written the day before. Again, when you've finished, put the rubber band around the pages. Do this for thirty days. At the end of thirty days, when you read the notes you've made, you'll be surprised to find you've made a very thorough analysis of yourself. If you've been honest with yourself, the result will be valuable.

Another method of self-analysis that has helped a lot of people is the Personality Report. Write it as you would a news story. Know how to write a news story? It's simple enough—in form, anyhow. It consists of the Five W's: Who, What, When, Where and Why. Write a short self-portrait, using each of the five W's as the basis of a paragraph. Tell yourself why you are fat, why you want to be thin, what you intend to do about it, even what you've learned about yourself in regard to your superfluous weight.

Perhaps these tests, though they may sound quite simple to you, will help you solve your own obesity problems. You may need more psychiatrical or psychological treatment. Your own state of mind, once you've had a medical examination, will determine that. Or your physician may be able to determine, immediately, if you need mental as well as physical treatment, or if he can give you necessary psychosomatic analysis. Certainly you need treatment—expert treatment you haven't been able to give yourself—or you wouldn't be fat. With all of the progress that has been made in medicine and science, you'd be very foolish not to take advantage of the best treatment you can get. After all, you are your own most valuable possession. To stay as well and as young as possible means making the best of yourself. By being slender and alert and well-balanced and good-looking, you are giving to the world your best self—and you will get the best in return. You can be practically anything you want to be, within reason—I'm not offering miracles—if you throw away the shackles of an Inferiority Complex, a false covering of fat and vague longings and wishes, and start doing the things you really want to do. Looking and feeling well will give you confidence, self-possession and, if you manage right, contentment.

You will get thin—and stay thin—only when you have conquered self. You must know yourself—gain a feeling of relaxation and peace, a freedom from fear. If you fed secure, you won't have to eat the wrong foods, or too much food. No secure person actually craves food! You will eat—and enjoy—foods that are good for you. If you are starved for affection, you may believe it is food that you want. Get the affection! Don't settle for food! You can help nature reduce you to your perfect proportions if you conquer self. Self-discipline is the only way to weight perfection, if you want to get—and stay— slender. The real secret of thinking yourself thin.

CHAPTER 10

You eat your
cake and have it

IF YOU'VE READ everything I've written up to now, you've
learned probably as much as you can learn about yourself and your own mental and physical condition in regard
to overweight without more expert advice than I—or
anyone else—can give you without a personal examination. And that is what you need, now.

If you're following my advice on thinking yourself
thin, you know that you need the best professional guidance you can get if you want to get thin, and stay thin. I
can give you general ideas, and shall try to give them to
you, but without a personal analysis, you'll not be able
to do too well. My rule for thinking yourself thin includes an examination by your own physician.

If I were you, I'd finish reading all of this first, for
three reasons. You'll understand the subject of obesity
and food much better. You'll be able to explain to your
own physician what sort of an examination you want and
need. And, best of all, you'll be able to understand and
follow his directions—and mine, too.

So, read this to the end. Then take the book to your
doctor. If he hasn't seen it, it may interest him. If he

has seen it, and knows that you have read it and understand it, he'll be able to discuss your own condition with you much more intelligently.

Remember that most physicians today are far too busy curing people who are very ill to bother too much about obesity, if it does not seem too serious to them. All obesity is serious—to the person who is overweight. But the average physician hasn't taken time to devote himself to a study of overweight. But there are physicians who specialize in obesity. There are a number of these physicians in every city. Dr. Sidney M. Schnittke of New York specializes in obesity cases. He is also the physician in attendance at the Du Barry Success School. Dr. M. B. Feiner of the Bronx has an excellent reputation for reducing hundreds of women. There are dozens of other physicians who specialize in obesity. But even these doctors cannot perform miracles. They can examine you, and prescribe for you if you need special treatment. They can tell you about your own condition. Your own family physician, even if he is not an obesity specialist, can give you a thorough examination—and expert advice. Then, with his specialized advice for you, and the help of this book, you'll be on the right track toward slenderness.

For, after you have learned why you are fat, you must realize that in order to be thin there are certain things that you must do. You must get your body and mind in good condition—whether that means treatment by a physician and/or a psychiatrist. You must do a certain amount of exercise. And—and oh, how I hate to say that awful four-letter word—you must—here

I go—*diet !* There's no way to avoid it. Your doctor may give you certain things to help you. The exercise will undoubtedly firm your muscles, and make your dieting a bit easier—and you'll look better. But diet is the basis of every obesity cure. It needn't be a horrible diet. In fact, I have some very good ideas about diet that I believe will help you. But diet is indicated!

Dr. Feiner told me, "Ninety-eight per cent of obesity is based on bad eating habits," and Dr. Schnittke prescribes medication when needed—plus a high-protein diet. You'll hear more about diet and exercise—but make up your mind, here, that you'll have to accept them. The exercises I advise are mild and painless—but they are exercises. And the diet—though some of it is pleasant —is still diet. A lot of my recipes which have never been published before—they are my own invention—are really substitutes for whipped cream and sour cream and luscious high-calorie desserts. The salad dressings I'll tell you about are good—but not nearly as good as some of the non-diet dressings. Cream sauces are out—and the substitutes may not be as pleasing to you, in the beginning. But you'll eat well—and live well. You won't starve, and you won't be hungry. But getting thin will be a real task. And staying thin will be somewhat of a task, too. I don't mind it at all! Only occasionally do I cast an envious eye at a window full of forbidden foodstuffs. But Pd rather have my figure and feel the way I do than be fat and wobbly—and eat chocolates. You've got to choose, and I've made my choice. You are starting not only a diet, but a new outlook—a new way of living.

Edwin L. Baron, who, according to the *New York Herald Tribune,* is a stage performer and holds a degree in psychology, has been using hypnosis successfully to cut women's weight. He puts his "patients" to sleep, telling them they will no longer want fattening foods when they awaken. He says he can cure appetites for tobacco and liquor, too. You don't need hypnosis! You can convince yourself of your need for high-protein, rich-in-vitamin foods, and cultivate an understanding of them and a taste for them on your own.

The late Dr. Herbert Vermilye reduced many patients by making them learn the foods that were good for them, and planning with them a sensible diet of fruit, vegetables, meat, milk and eggs that they liked and understood.

Dr. Albert C. Santy, one of New York's fine physicians, who has helped his patients on diets lose many, many pounds, believes that you can't say to a patient that he must cut out certain foods—even if he should go without them. That will just make him crave the foods all the more. Dr. Santy believes, with all of the other physicians I spoke to, that his patients should go on a high-protein diet. He limits them as to calories, gives appetite depressors, explains about foods, and then tells them:

"Go ahead! Eat what you like! But you must eat very small quantities of the foods that are not for you. If you go on the way you've been going, you cannot get thin.

If you must go on a mild eating binge once in a while, that is up to you. But you must make up for it the following day."

He told me about one patient who swore she kept to her 1,000-calorie diet. But she didn't lose a pound 1 When he questioned her at length, he found she had about ten alcoholic drinks a day. Someone had told her that alcohol wasn't fattening! When she followed Dr. Santy's advice and began counting her alcoholic calories, three things happened: She practically stopped drinking. Her health improved. She lost weight. She wouldn't stop drinking entirely and, as she was not an alcoholic, it wasn't necessary. But, by eating the proper foods, and thinking about what she was trying to do, she decreased her appetite for both food and liquor. Now she has a good figure, is in excellent health, and eats and drinks just the things that are good for her.

You see, the old saw, "You can't eat your cake and have it," was never written for the fat person. For, unfortunately, we fat people can eat our cake and have it. That's the trouble. When we do eat cake, we do have it—forever. This is to advise you that you can't eat your cake at all. Not the cake you're accustomed to, anyhow.

What to do 'til the doctor comes? Read this book. Keep up your notes on your weight and on your own diet. When you go to your doctor, after you've finished reading this, take with you all of your notes. Show him your weight. Show him what you've been eating. That will be a better introduction than most of his patients bring him. In fact, usually, he has to ask diet questions. And receive those good old answers, "Why Doctor, I eat hardly anything 1 Less than any of my friends. I eat like a bird!"

Think how pleased your doctor will be when you hand him your notes—a full list of the foods you've eaten for weeks, with their caloric values written next to them. You'll put in the caloric values before too long, now. You'll have the full diagram of your regulation diet— for your own information. He'll have it—for his. And he'll be able to tell, at once, what you are eating that is wrong for you, and how you'll have to change your diet to suit his rules—and mine. I have an idea they'll be a lot alike, varied only by your own personal needs. I think he'll be grateful because you come to him with an intelligent outlook—and intelligent preparation.

How often you'll have to visit your doctor is up to him, and up to your own physical condition. It may be— and quite possibly will be—that only a very few visits may be necessary. One good physical examination, plus a diet and any necessary medication, plus a check-up to see that you are following instructions, may be all you need. Or you may need a whole lot more. A complete course at a gymnasium or beauty school, or many visits to your doctor.

Here is what you should want—and get—at the first visit to your physician. You'll find that obesity is no longer a mysterious disease, and that its permanent cure does not consist of clipping diets out of newspapers or magazines or passing along secret advice, but is as scientific as anything can be, these days.

Your examination will depend on your condition, and on your physician. Although it will differ in some respects, it will have certain definite aspects.

First, there will probably be questions about your history, and your family's history, and questions with regard to such illnesses as hypertension, diabetes and fevers, the weight of other members of your family, and your own weight at birth and during childhood. The doctor will ask you about how long you sleep, if you use tobacco, drugs, alcohol and tea and coffee.

He will then ask you about your eating habits—and be pleased when you produce the full data on how much you've eaten during the past weeks, and can tell him exactly about your food habits. He will also ask about fluid intake and how much salt you use.

Next, there will probably be questions about your emotional life. You've already analyzed your emotions, I'm sure, when you read the pages that went before this. The information you gathered about yourself will be valuable on your visit to your doctor.

There will undoubtedly be questions about menstrual history, if you're a woman, and questions about your thyroid condition, based on your ability to stand heat and cold, the condition of your hair and nails, and even if your perspiration is normal.

If your doctor gives you a thorough examination—and I hope he will—he will examine your body to see if you have one of the glandular types of obesity.

Sometimes an X-ray examination is necessary. Possible tumors, hypothyroidism and other illnesses can be discovered by X-ray examination.

A routine examination will be made, of course, of your heart. And your blood pressure will be taken, so that, if you have hypertension, you can be placed on a salt-free diet, and other diet necessary for your condition can be prescribed. At one time, normal blood pressure was supposedly 100 plus your age. Now physicians believe that the perfect blood pressure is much lower, and they pay special attention to it in regard to obesity. Blood pressure is "the pressure exerted by the blood on the walls of the vessels in which it is flowing." A lot of factors influence blood pressure, including the force of the heartbeat, the elasticity of the walls of the blood vessels, and the secretions of ductless glands. The physician wraps the bag around the arm, uses a stethoscope to determine systolic and diastolic pressure. Systolic pressure, from 20 to 70 years of age, should average from 120 to 138 degrees, and diastolic pressure may range from 79 to 89 degrees. A slight variation is unimportant, except to the physician, who may learn a lot about your condition from it. 120 degrees, at 20 years of age, plus half a point a year, is a lot more accurate than the older method for systolic pressure. High blood pressure can be an indication of a dozen illnesses, including neuroses.

Your basal metabolism is important. While most obese people, in spite of their preconceived notions, have a normal metabolic rate, it still must be taken, in case there is hypothyroidism. The patient eats a light meal the night before, one containing very little protein. He should rest before the test and not be nervous or worried. The basal metabolism test is the method of measuring how much oxygen is used during an hour. Tests usually last about ten minutes, during which the patient breathes through a rubber mouthpiece from a tank containing a measured amount of air. When the thyroid hormone supply is inadequate, the rate of oxygen used is reduced.

A chemical examination of the blood should be made. From a blood count, a doctor can learn if there are too few red or white corpuscles or platelets, and this tells the presence of disease. The hemoglobin test shows how much coloring matter there is in the blood—whether the blood cells are round and normal or distorted. Often, people who are too fat have anemia—the amount of hemoglobin in the blood is reduced below normal. Most people do not know that anemia and obesity can go together—but they can. The physician knows what medicine is indicated, and the things he prescribes help the blood, but do not add weight. It is necessary to check for a low basal metabolic rate determination. The determination of the glucose content of the blood is usually necessary, too.

A glucose tolerance test is important for the diagnosis of defects of carbohydrate metabolism. And a urine test is necessary, too. The normal person shows traces of sugar one hour after eating, and sometimes shows a slight trace after two hours. A poor sugar tolerance is present if glucose is found in large amounts, or continues into the third hour.

Sometimes other gland tests are made, though these are not often considered necessary.

These tests determine if the patient has obesity of the endogenous or glandular type—which is rare, and even then the glandular defect is practically always only an indirect cause of obesity. Reduction of weight without diet is almost impossible in glandular cases, even when hormones are given. The exogenous form of obesity can be cured by diet alone—and without glandular treatment.

Doctors will prescribe thyroid or other glandular drugs, when they are indicated. And most doctors will prescribe drugs that are either metabolic stimulants or appetite depressors. Benzedrine sulfate or dexedrine, or other appetite depressors, sometimes help control the desire to eat, or give a sense of wellbeing.

Diuretics are often used—especially in the beginning of a diet, to encourage the patient. These cause the excretion of a few pounds of water, and are often used if there is a great deal of water retention. If this is followed by a water-restricted diet, combined with salt restriction, a substantial reduction often results. Many people lose weight if less water and salt are used. Your doctor will tell you more about these.

Most doctors put their patients on a low-calorie diet, ranging from 6oo to 1,200 calories per day—and averaging around 1,000 calories—usually with a high protein content. Sometimes these diets consist of printed lists, which must be followed exactly. Other doctors believe that their patients have the intelligence to make up their own diets, when full directions as to food restrictions are given. Dr. Feiner tells me that, for the average patient, he prescribes a 1,000-calorie intake, limits fluid to four glasses per day, allows no fruit except stewed fruits, and orders mostly high-protein food, with a limited number of cocktails and highballs, but no beer or wine. He gives medicine when indicated. He has successfully reduced hundreds of people. No secrets, he says. Just common sense, appetite depressors, glandular treatment, when indicated, and a sensible diet of three low-calorie meals a day.

Dr. Schnittke advises a simple low-calorie, high-protein diet. I shall give this diet, as well as a number of other diets, in full, in subsequent chapters.

This is just to show you what happens when you visit your doctor for your important check-up. As soon as you find out just what is wrong with you—the reason for your obesity—you're ready to reduce. Your reduction will consist of whatever medicinal treatment is prescribed, plus the low-calorie diet.

Although you should not diet until you have received the go-ahead from your own physician, you may as well learn about food values, if you don't already know about them, so that you'll be ready to reduce, once you have had your examination.

In the meantime, go ahead with your weighing in at morning, and your food tabulations at night. You're to continue those, even after you are on your diet, you know. They are part of the Think Yourself Thin system.

CHAPTER II

Portrait of you

THIS IS A PORTRAIT of YOU. So, of course, it's one of the shortest pieces in the book. Just when you thought there was a fine chance to hear about yourself I

"I'm nothing like these cases you've told about," I can hear you say. "Or not much, anyhow. Why, they're neurotic, with all of their fears and illnesses and frustrations—their wishes to be taken care of, and their desires for escape. I'm perfectly all right! The only thing the matter with me is that I'm overweight. And I'm overweight simply because I love to eat good food.'[1]

Could be as simple as that. It's been proven to be as simple as that. As you say, you're in such good health that you digest your food so well that every extra calorie goes into fat. And you love to eat. You know good food and you want quite a lot of it. What can you do?

As if you didn't know I You can diet and lose weight. And combine the diet with the right exercises. But you hate to diet, and you loathe exercise. But you want to lose weight—want to be thin. What can you do? Well, of course, like all of the others, you can think yourself thin, too.

You can't think yourself thin, and keep on eating the way you have been eating. That much is certain. But you can think yourself thin, if you'll change your eating habits. And that doesn't mean you have to go on a bread-and-water, lamb-chop-and-pineapple or grapefruit-and-raw-salad regime, either. It does mean you have to change, first of all, your outlook, and second, your eating habits. Both hard jobs. Both possible, if you'll put your mind to it—if you'll actually think yourself thin.

Because this is a portrait of you, you who have good appetites and love to eat, I can draw a pretty accurate portrait of you—and what you've done, so far, and without too much success, to lose weight.

At some time or other you've probably gone to a doctor and got a diet from him. And carried the diet list—probably a printed or mimeographed list—around in your pocket, taking it out at mealtimes, and trying, for a few weeks, anyhow, to adhere to it. You probably lost quite a few pounds, while you kept to it. But you did it with your body—with your digestive organs—and without much of your mind. You wanted to be thin, but you didn't do anything serious about it. You lost the pounds—and perhaps your face grew too thin, and someone said, "You look awful!" And you didn't feel any too well—no energy at all. So you gave up THAT diet—and gained back all of the weight you lost, and perhaps a few pounds extra, for good measure.

Someone gave you a "magic" diet. They got it from a doctor, or from a friend, or out of a book. And you tried that for a while, and lost a few pounds—but some parties came along, or you got invited out to dinner, and the diet was so dull that you never went back to it.

Maybe you took thyroid. You'd be surprised at the number of normal people, who have nothing at all the matter with their metabolism, who take thyroid, thinking that a few grains of thyroid will work magic and turn them from being fat and flabby into being firm, young and slender. If you need thyroid, small doses of it will assist you in reaching normal weight—normal metabolism—but you'll have to diet while you're taking it. Thyroid, unless you need it, is useless, or worse than useless. In fact, it might upset your metabolism, and do real harm.

Perhaps you took one of the newer appetite destroyers, or appetite depressors. You probably took one that wasn't at all suitable for you, so it didn't depress your appetite at all. It may even have made you nervous. Or you may have taken the right one for you, and expected magic from it. Even if you do need—and take—an appetite depressor, all it will do is to take the edge off your appetite, or make you feel satisfied before you've eaten too much food.

You probably went in for strenuous exercise, at one time or another, hating every minute of it, and gaining a tremendous appetite so that you ate more than ever, and gained weight, instead of losing it.

Undoubtedly, you once went in for massage, if you've been fat for a long time. The masseuse came regularly, and you stretched out luxuriously and got pummeled and squashed. If you didn't diet along with it, you probably didn't lose at all. If you did diet with it, you probably lost a little, and gained all the weight back, the minute you stopped the massage. I hate to tell you this, but you probably know it, anyhow. Do you know who was reduced most by that massage? Why, of course, the person who did all the work—the masseuse who got fine exercise while you lay prone! Massage is fine. But it only helps—does not cause much actual reduction.

You may have taken one of the beauty courses—fine, in themselves, if you put your mind to it—and thought yourself thin, along with the course. In fact, if you did that, you don't need this at all. But more than likely, the course never went below the surface of your mind. You skimmed over it—and, therefore, as soon as it was over, there you were, gaining weight again. I have known people who were permanently helped by various beauty courses—but they used their brains with their treatments. I've known others who have lost temporarily—and then went back to their previous weight, once they finished the "course" and mentally went back to their old ways.

You may have bought a book—and gone in heavily for yogurt, wheat germ and black molasses, helping the manu-facturers of these products quite a lot, and yourself very little. These products, along with other health foods, are excellent in their ways. Some of them are moderately low in calories. Others are extremely high in calories—and greatly overrated in what they have to offer. More about those later on, too. Because of your lack of food knowledge, these foods did not get the right place in your diet program. You ate too many calories of them—and

wondered why you didn't reduce. They're supposed to reduce you, aren't they? Taken in proper proportions, at
proper times, they're all right in any well-balanced diet.
You must learn when, and how, and why to use them.

You say, "Why, I do diet! I've given up practically all
potatoes and gravies and bread and butter and rich desserts, and I haven't lost a pound." And you don't know
that potatoes and bread, in moderation—the right moderation—are not especially fattening. And that the nibbles
you have with cocktails and between meals give you a
lot more fat-forming calories than bread or potatoes
could ever do.

You say, "I eat a lot of fruit and vegetables—and still
I don't reduce." Too much fruit and the wrong vegetables, without enough protein, are fattening. You'll
learn more about fruit and vegetables—if you care about
learning. Just stick to this and see!

Or you shrug your shoulders and say, "How on earth
can I reduce!" And give one of these four reasons. 1. You
live alone, and it's mighty hard to reduce when you're
alone. 2. You live with a big family—or with one other
person—and it's mighty hard to reduce when other people are around. 3. You live at home, and it's mighty hard
to reduce when you eat every meal at home. 4. You eat
in restaurants, and isn't it practically impossible to reduce
when you eat out?

You know as well as I do that these excuses are just
that—excuses. Alibis. And not very good ones. If you
make up your mind to reduce, these difficulties will just

add fun to the reduction. Extra hazards. Things you can overcome.

You can't reduce permanently by following blindly a bit of printed paper, whether it's a vague or definite menu, scattered or concise directions. You can reduce only if you understand what reduction is all about, and, understanding it, follow the knowledge you have gained. In other words, think yourself thin.

The method? As if you haven't guessed, by now.

First, you should have found out what you weigh. You should have found out what you should weigh. Which gives you, simple as anything, the amount you should lose. Your rate of loss had best be determined by your own physician—and your own health.

Second, you should have your doctor's advice on your own reduction problem. He'll probably suggest a special diet. He may give you—and probably will give you—an appetite depressor. He'll undoubtedly tell you how many calories a day you ought to eat. It will probably be around 1,000 calories, while you're losing weight, and a far more liberal allowance, once you've reached the weight that is perfect for you. The amount you'll eat, even then, will undoubtedly be less than you eat now. You'll learn to compare this with your present diet.

Third, you must learn about foods and their values. Not only their calories, but their carbohydrate, their protein and their fat content. And you must learn how much of these foods are right for you, and in what proportion.

Fourth, you must learn about the vitamin and mineral contents of food. And you'll find out, likely as not, in these days of buying foods that have been picked a long time before they reach you, or which have been canned or even frozen, that they have lost part of their vitamin value, and must be supplemented by vitamins. Your own doctor will suggest a vitamin supplement—something to take the place of the lost vitamins, due to our present mode of living, when this is necessary.

Next, you must learn to choose your own diet. To choose, from the foods that are right for you, the foods that you can eat three or four times a day. With the knowledge, you'll be able to make up your own diet—a diet you can follow easily, because you've chosen it from the foods you like, within the classes of foods that are open to you. No longer will you have to accept, blindly, anyone's printed menu or printed diet list, unless you prefer it to your own. You'll know what you're eating and why!

After that, you must learn to forget about food, except when you are ordering it or preparing it—or eating it. In other words, a lot of fat is brought about because of a concentration on food. We think about foods, so we want to eat—and when we want to eat, we do eat; and when we eat, we eat too much—and get fat. If we throw the thought of food out of our minds, except when the thoughts should be there, we'll still eat well—but only when we should. And we'll get thin. Thinking yourself thin includes forgetting about foods when you shouldn't be thinking about them. This takes a strong character— but thinking yourself thin isn't a process for weaklings.

You must be interested in other things, things outside of yourself—so interested in them that food is just an incidental part of your life, not the main part of it at all. I hope you'll always enjoy eating—that dining will still be an important pleasure. But I hope you'll turn your mind outside, to a hundred other things, so that food will be just one thing you'll have on your mind. Life will be far more interesting when food takes its rightful place. Eating is far too important to the average person who weighs too much. He substitutes other pleasures for food —even if he doesn't always admit it. And even when he does, food is still too great a part of his life. Keep on enjoying your dinners. But don't make them the big thing in your life. There's music and art and the theatre and the movies and radio and television and books and science and your family and friends, and affection and love. When those—and your work and other personal interests —all occupy your mind in their right proportions, then food will take its rightful place, too. See what I mean about thinking yourself thin?

CHAPTER 12

Food for thought

HOW MUCH DO YOU KNOW ABOUT FOODS? Not too much, I'd like to wager, even if you have been dieting and reading about diet. I'm always amazed, when I find out how little people know—how little I knew when I began to learn about foods—about thinking yourself thin. Even now, each day I learn something new. And as new food discoveries are made, I hope I'll go on learning new things. So I can tell you what scientists and specialists believe— as of today. Tomorrow, the newspapers may contain new facts about food—even new ways to grow thin.

Today, the high-protein diet is considered by far the best diet for weight reduction, and for the maintenance of correct weight, once the reduction is complete. Certainly, every diet requires some carbohydrates and some fat—and all good diets contain those in the right proportion, as well as vitamins and minerals. By lessening your carbohydrate and fat intake, and increasing your protein intake, you lose weight, providing the right amounts of the right foods are eaten. Of course, water and salt are impo-

In the stomach, proteins are broken down by pepsin and hydrochloric acid to proteoses and peptones, and, finally, in the intestines, to amino acids. There are about twenty-two amino acids—and ten of these are essential to health. Some very good proteins contain all of the amino acids. These are perfect for health and reduction. Others are incomplete, and do not contain all of the amino acids, though they are good, too.

Proteins are the "building blocks" of the body, though that terminology, of course, is inexact, as the body isn't a fixed, solid structure. The value of protein is determined by the completeness with which it supplies all the amino acids needed to build the body.

If a person gets enough proteins, his body has a nitrogen balance. If the proteins do not provide enough, then he is in negative balance. A nitrogen equilibrium is a real factor in a good diet—and can be attained even if a person is losing weight, if enough protein is taken.

The chief function of carbohydrates in nutrition is to give energy. They are the most rapidly utilized of all food materials. When too much carbohydrates are taken into the body, they form fat. If not enough are taken, the body draws on its own tissues—and a person loses weight.

Fat, as part of the diet, was considered, in the past, to have only high caloric value. But fat also gives energy and provides substances necessary for animal economy. Some fat is needed in every diet.

However, protein not only provides building blocks. It does more than that. It stimulates the metabolism so much that instead of 100 calories, there will be a rise to 130 calories. This is known as "specific dynamic action" —and means that you may eat more protein and not gain, but actually lose weight.

Today, practically all authorities recognize the need for a liberal protein diet, especially in reduction. The "low-protein era" was introduced by Chittenden, following his experiments with a group of young men, and is now considered to be without too much value because there was no "control" group upon whom the experiment could be measured, and because his experiments were too short. Further experiments by many physicians, both in reduction and in regular diets, have proved the value of high protein in every good diet, for the maintenance of continued health, as well as for weight reduction.

To reduce weight, an obese person must burn his own body fat. It's as simple as that. He must eat himself up! A bit cannibalistic? I'm afraid so. But it's the only way to lose weight. Eating less—and increasing food utilization by exercise. And, while dieting, care must be taken against protein loss, by increasing the protein intake; against mineral and vitamin deficiency, by eating the right foods and taking extra vitamins when necessary; and against hunger, by eating satisfactory and satisfying foods.

The protein foods are the first ones to be considered in a reduction diet. No one is supposed to live exclusively on proteins—though people have lived on them without ill effects. Some people say that too many proteins cause acidosis, but you needn't worry about that—you'll undoubtedly eat enough other foods to prevent this.

Meats are among the best source of good proteins. Explorers have lived on meat alone, and have remained in good health, year after year. And our ancestors are supposed to have lived on meat—raw meat at that—and lived long and survived hardships. Today, we'll cook our foods—even if we destroy a part of the proteins. And we'll combine them with other foods, for a balanced diet.

The internal meats were considered the best sources of protein. They are still good. But all meats contain complete proteins—all of the amino acids. The best meats for good protein value are liver, kidneys, sweetbreads, brains, heart, lean beef, chicken, tongue, lamb chops, steak, turkey, stews, roast beef, pork, veal and tripe. The dark meat of poultry has a slightly higher protein value than the light meat, but both are excellent.

All dairy products are high in protein, though, of course, on a reduction diet, it really can't matter to you whether or not cream or the cheeses that are high in fat contain protein, too, for you can't have them. Luckily, there are excellent dairy products which have a low fat content, and are high in protein as well. These are buttermilk, skimmed milk, cottage cheese and pot cheese. These will form an important part of your high-protein diet.

For a long time, now, it's been thought that many types of heart disorders were due to a high cholesterol content in the diet. This was based on the fact that cholesterol-like deposits have been found in the coronary blood vessels, the occlusion of which causes hearts to fail. It was found that people who suffered from coronary occlusion often ate foods high in cholesterol. However, other people ate the same foods and suffered no heart trouble. Now, they find that the trouble is a lack of the factor necessary for the proper metabolism of cholesterol. Dr. Ancel Keys, Director of the University of Minnesota Laboratory of Physical Hygiene, conducted a study, with 482 men as subjects, and found that the body produces cholesterol despite the foods you eat. He found that eating dairy products, meats, and eggs—all high in cholesterol content—does not lead to increased cholesterol in the blood. And that even foods that contain no cholesterol may raise the cholesterol level of the blood. By reducing the consumption of high-protein foods, the diet lacks essential nutrients. Nutrition scientists are agreed that an adequate diet should include dairy foods, fruits, meats, fish, eggs, vegetables and cereals.

Practically all seafoods are high in protein. By omitting the fatty fish, you still have a large variety to chose from. These can form the main dish of a meal—or an excellent first course. High in protein are oysters, clams, shrimps, salmon and tuna fish—when served without too much oil—and practically every kind of fresh fish, both from fresh and salt water. These allow a varied and well-flavored diet, even when limited to non-fattening foods.

All nuts are high in protein. The only trouble is that they are high in fat content, too. They may be substituted, occasionally, for meat, or used in a diet that is poor in protein and fat, but they can't be eaten in large quantities with other fattening foods. Peanuts—which are not nuts, but a vegetable, they tell me—are high in protein value. So are almonds, pecans, walnuts, pistaschios and pignolias. Go slow with these, though 1

Many vegetables that are high in protein are, alas, fattening, too, so they cannot be eaten in large quantities. The highest in protein are all types of soya beans. Next are lentils, corn and lima beans. Peas and potatoes contain proteins, too. All green vegetables contain valuable proteins, vitamins and minerals, give bulk, and are needed in every reduction diet.

Bread is valuable for its protein content. But too much bread is fattening. However, even on a get-thin diet, some bread is good—and even necessary. Excellent high-protein breads, rich in gluten and soya flours, are for sale in most health stores. Regulation whole wheat bread, and even ordinary "store bought" white bread, with added vitamin content, is good in reduction diets, when limited in quantity. High-protein spaghetti, available in health stores, too, is a good addition to the reduction diet—when not used too frequently, or in too large quantities. Toast is no better on a reduction diet than bread. It's just bread with the moisture removed.

Eggs are very high in protein. When cooked without added fat, they are among the best sources of protein. Gelatin is a good—but incomplete—protein.

You will, of course, avoid practically all fats on your new diet. I'll give fat substitutes in the recipe section. This is just the first reminder of what you can and can't eat. Complete tables, giving the contents of all the foods you'll probably care about eating, will show you even more definitely why you should avoid fats. Fats, of course, include salad oils, olive oils, cooking fats, fats on meat, all fried food, except as stated later, gravies, all rich sauces, avocados, nuts—except as an occasional meat substitute—ripe olives, all pastries, cakes, cookies, rich desserts, candies, jellies and marmalades.

What else can you eat, then, except the high proteins? Oh, lots of things! As much of the fruits and vegetables from Group I, the 3% carbohydrate foods, as you wish —within reason, of course. They are fine for you. Generous servings of foods from Group 2, the 6% carbohydrates. A limited amount from Group 3, the 9% carbohydrates, and Group 5, the 15% carbohydrates. But you must avoid all foods in Group 6, except, of course, garlic, horseradish and other flavoring, and, occasionally, potatoes. The highest carbohydrate foods in the miscellaneous group must not be included in any reduction diets.

Later on, you'll learn more about combining these foods, and using them to the best advantage. This is your first "lesson" in food values. I hope you won't find it too difficult, for there's a lot more to follow! You see, I'd really like you to know a lot about food values. Only in that way can you think yourself thin, so that you'll get— and stay—as thin as you ought to be, and enjoy the process as much as anyone can enjoy anything that does mean a definite sacrifice of some of the good things of living. If you give up foods with your eyes open, and know why you avoid them, the avoiding isn't nearly so difficult.

These lists are from the U.S. Department of Agriculture. The canned products, as noted, must be without additional sugar. "W.P." means water-packed, that is, canned with water only, and "J.P." means juice-packed, with the juice of the fruit included, but no extra sugar added. Of course, you may add a sugar substitute, one of the non-fattening ones—more about those later—if you like a sweeter fruit. I know I do. Here, then, are your first lists.

Group I (3 *per cent carbohydrate*)

Asparagus, fresh.
Asparagus, canned, including
   sieved.
Asparagus-bean sprouts, fresh.
Bamboo shoots, fresh.
Basella, fresh.
Beans, green and wax, canned,
   including sieved.
Bean sprouts (from mung
   beans), fresh.
Beet greens, fresh.
Broccoli, fresh.
Cabbage, fresh.
Cabbage, Chinese, fresh.
Cauliflower, fresh.
Cauliflower, canned.
Celery, fresh.
Celery, canned, sieved.
Chard, fresh.
Chayote, leaves, fresh.
Chicory, leaves, fresh.
Corn salad, fresh.
Cress, garden, fresh.

Cucumbers, fresh.
Dock, fresh.
Endive, fresh.
Escarole, fresh.
Fennel, fresh.
"French endive," fresh.
Lettuce, fresh.
Mustard greens, fresh.
Orach, garden, fresh.
Orach, Peruvian, fresh.
Pokeberry or poke shoots,
   fresh.
Purslane, fresh.
Quinoa, fresh.
Radishes, fresh.
Rhubarb, fresh.
Rhubarb, canned, w. p.
Rutabaga tops, fresh.
Sauerkraut, fresh.
Sauerkraut, canned.
Seakale, fresh.
Sorrel, fresh.
Spinach, fresh.

Spinach, canned, including sieved.
Spinach, New Zealand, fresh.
Squash, summer, fresh.
Taro shoots, fresh.
Tomatoes, fresh.
Tomatoes, canned.

Tomato juice, fresh.
Tomato juice, canned.
Turnip tops, fresh.
Udo shoots, fresh.
Vegetable marrow, fresh.
Vinespinach, fresh.
Water cress, fresh.

Group II (6 per cent carbohydrate)

Amaranth, fresh.
Anserine, fresh.
Beans, hyacinth-bean, pods, fresh.
Beans, scarlet runner, green pods, fresh.
Beans, snap, green and wax, fresh.
Blackberries, canned, w. p.
Borage, fresh.
Cantaloupe.
Carrots, canned, including sieved.
Celery root or celeriac, fresh.
Chayote, fruit, fresh.
Chives, fresh.
Collards, fresh.
Dandelion greens, fresh.
Dasheen, leaves, and stems, fresh.
Eggplant, fresh.
Gooseberries, canned, w. p.
Jew's mallow, fresh.
Kale, fresh.
Kohlrabi, fresh.
Lambsquarters, fresh

Leeks, fresh.
Melons, honeydew, casaba, and Spanish, fresh.
Muskmelons, fresh.
Nettle, fresh.
Okra, fresh.
Onions, Welsh, fresh.
Palmetto or palmetto cabbage, fresh.
Parsley, fresh.
Peaches, canned, w. p.
Peppers, green and red, fresh.
Pimientos, canned.
Plums, excluding prunes, canned, w. p.
Pumpkin, fresh.
Pumpkin and squash, canned.
Salad-rocket, fresh.
Soybeans, green shelled, fresh.
Soybean sprouts, fresh.
Squash, cushaw, fresh.
Squash, winter, fresh.
Strawberries, fresh.
Strawberries, canned, w. p. and j. p.
Strawberry juice, fresh.

Sweetpotato tops, fresh.   Turnips, fresh.
Taro, leaves and stems, fresh.   Watermelon, fresh.

Group HI (9 per cent carbohydrate)

Applesauce, canned, unsweet-   Lemon juice, fresh.
    ened.   Lemon juice, canned.
Apricots, canned, w. p.   Limes, fresh.
Artichokes, globe or French,   Limes, sweet, fresh.
    fresh.   Lime juice, fresh
Asparagus-beans, pods, fresh.   Loganberries, canned w. p.
Beets, fresh.   Loganberry juice, fresh.
Beets, canned, including   Mamey, fresh.
    sieved.   Mammee apple, fresh.
Blackberries, fresh.   Onions, fresh.
Blackberries, canned, j. p.   Oranges, mandarin type,
Blackberry juice, fresh.   fresh.
Blueberries, canned, w. p.   Orange juice, mandarin type,
    and j. p.   fresh.
Brussels sprouts, fresh.   Papayas, fresh.
Cape-gooseberry, fresh.   Parsley, Hamburg, fresh.
Carrots, fresh.   Peaches, canned, j. p.
Cherries, red and white,   Pears, canned, w. p.
    canned, w. p.   Peas, fresh (very young).
Chervil, fresh.   Peas, canned, including sieved.
Cranberries, fresh.   Peas, sugar peas, green pods,
Currants, fresh.   fresh.
Currant juice, fresh.   Poha, fresh.
Gingerroot, fresh.   Pricklypear, fresh.
Gooseberries, fresh.   Prunes, canned, w. p.
Grapefruit, fresh.   Quince juice, fresh.
Grapefruit, canned, w. p.   Raspberries, canned, w. p.
    and j. p.   Rutabagas, fresh.
Grapefruit juice, fresh.   Tangerines, fresh.
Groundcherry, fresh.   Tangerine juice, fresh.
Lemons, fresh.

Group IV (12 *per cent carbohydrate*)

Apple juice, fresh.
Applesauce, canned, j. p.
Apricots, fresh.
Apricots, canned, j. p.
Apricots, canned, sieved,
  unsweetened.
Beans, lima, green, canned.
Cherries, sour, fresh.
Cherries, red and white,
  canned, j. p.
Crab apple juice, fresh.
Feijoa, fresh.
Figs, canned, w. p.
Grapefruit juice, canned,
  unsweetened.
Grapes, canned, w. p.
Guavas, fresh.
Kumquats, fresh.
Lambsquarters, Algerian,
  fresh.
Loganberries, fresh.
Loganberries, canned, j. p.
Loquats, fresh.
Mulberries, fresh.
Oranges, fresh.

Oranges, Seville or sour,
fresh.
Orange juice, fresh.
Orange juice, canned.
Peaches, fresh.
Peaches, canned, sieved,
unsweetened.
Peach juice, fresh.
Pears, canned, j. p.
Pineapple, fresh.
Pineapple, canned, w. p.
Pineapple juice, fresh.
Pineapple juice, canned.
Pitanga, fresh.
Plums, excluding prunes,
fresh.
Quinces, fresh
Raspberries, fresh.
Raspberries, canned, j. p.
Raspberry juice, fresh.
Rose apple, fresh.
Soybeans, dry seeds.
Surinam cherry or pitanga,
fresh.

Group V (15 *per cent carbohydrate*)

Apples, fresh.
Beans, broadbeans, green
  shelled.
Beans, red kidney, canned.
Black-salsify, fresh.
Blueberries, fresh.

Blueberry juice, fresh.
Cherries, black, canned, w. p.
Corn, fresh (very young).
Grapes, fresh.
Huckleberries, fresh.
Huckleberry juice, fresh.

Jerusalem artichokes, tubers,
    fresh.
Mangos, fresh.
Nectarines, fresh.
Oca, fresh.
Onions, top onions, fresh.
Papaws, fresh.

Parsnips, fresh.
Pears, fresh.
Peas, fresh (medium mature).
Pineapple, canned, j. p.
Salsify, fresh.
Shallot, fresh.
Vegetable-oyster or salsify,
    fresh.

Group VI (18 *per cent carbohydrate)*

Beans, baked, canned.
Carissa or Natal plum, fresh.
Chayote, roots, fresh.
Cherries, sweet, fresh.
Cherries, black, canned, j. p.
Corn, sweet, canned.
Crab apples, fresh.
Figs, fresh.
Garlic, fresh.
Granadilla, purple, fresh.
Grape juice, fresh or bottled.
Haws, scarlet, fresh.

Horseradish, fresh.
Natal plum, fresh.
Passion fruit, fresh.
Persimmons, Japanese.
Pomegranates, fresh.
Potatoes, fresh.
Prunes, canned, j. p.
Prune juice, canned.
Sapodilla, fresh.
Sapota, fresh.
Waternut, tuber, fresh.

Miscellaneous Group (*high carbohydrate)*

Apples, dried.
Apricots, dried.
Asparagus-beans, dry.
Bananas, dried.
Bananas, fresh
Beans, broadbeans, dry.
Beans, kidney or common,
    dry.
Beans, lima, fresh.

Beans, lima, dry.
Beans, mung, dry.
Black-eyed peas, dry.
Burdock, fresh.
Cherimoya, fresh.
Cherries, maraschino, canned.
Chickpeas, dry.
Corn, fresh (medium mature
    and old).

Corn, dry, sweet, and field.
Cowpeas, fresh, green shelled.
Cowpeas, dry.
"Currants," dried.
Dasheen, tubers, fresh.
Dates, fresh and dried.
Figs, dried.
Fruits, canned in syrup (all kinds).
Garbanzo peas, dry.
Jujubes, fresh and dried.
Lentils, dry, whole and split.
Litchi fruit, dried.
Marmalade plum, fresh.
Peaches, dried.
Pears, dried.
Peas, fresh (mature).

Peas, dry, whole and split.
Persimmons, native, fresh.
Plantain, or baking banana, fresh.
Prunes, fresh.
Prunes, canned, sieved.
Prunes, dried.
Raisins, dried.
Sapote, fresh.
Sugar-apple, fresh.
Sweetpotatoes, fresh.
Sweetpotatoes, canned.
Sweetsop, fresh.
Taro, tubers, fresh.
Tomato catsup.
Yams, winged, fresh.

CHAPTER 13

Those vitamins!

You MAY AS WELL BE WARNED. This is the dullest part of this book on thinking yourself thin, it seems to me. How on earth can anyone make a vitamin interesting! I've never seen it done.

Of course I could omit this chapter altogether. But it wouldn't be fair to you. As a matter of fact, you really should know about vitamins. Without knowing about them you'll never actually understand food values, or know which foods to select for your own health. If you really want to think yourself thin—and if you've come along this far, I really think you do—you can just take this rather bitter pill along with the rest. I'll do my best to make it as brief and as instructive as possible—so please don't skip.

And how are your lists getting on? Think I forgot them ? Not at all! You can't think yourself thin without them. Every morning, you're supposed to weigh yourself—and then write down your weight. And every night you are—I hope—writing down everything you've eaten, against the time—not too far off now—when you're going

124

to check your list against what you ought to be eating—your own method of getting the correct diet for you.

Perhaps you're doing the Thirty Day Analysis, too, though you may not need that at all. But you do need the weight and the diet notes. I mean that, too!

And now I can't keep away from those vitamins another minute. You've heard so much about vitamins that you don't need a formal introduction, I'm sure. Vitamins are nutritive substances of which seemingly ridiculously small amounts are needed, but which can influence health and well-being to a remarkable extent. Animals get their nourishment from plants and the flesh of other animals. When these are too highly refined or purified or changed, diseases can result. Important factors are frequently lacking in purified and processed foods. By becoming too civilized we have laid ourselves open to ills. For too long a time we did away with too many vitamins and minerals. A new era was introduced when this fact was discovered.

As you probably know, the Japanese Navy, on old sailing vessels, was saved from beriberi by dietary changes. This was followed by experiments in the Dutch Indies. Not until 1913 did E. V. McCullum and M. Davis find that animals fed upon purified foodstuffs failed in normal growth, but that when rice polishings, egg yolk and other vitamins were added, normalcy was attained almost immediately. The discovery of Vitamin A was followed by Vitamin B and the other known vitamins. New vitamins and new food elements are still being frequently discovered by scientists.

The average person can find enough vitamins in well-selected foods. But people on diets frequently have to add supplementary vitamins, when recommended by their physicians. All vitamins help toward health and energy. Six vitamins have been discovered to have definite usage. Several more have been isolated, but their exact need has not yet been determined.

Vitamin A—the fat-soluble vitamin—is the yellow pigment in carotene, and chlorophyll in green plants, among other things. This valuable vitamin is needed for growth, for vitality, to help protect one against disease by building up resistance. It is good for the eyes, and helps actual vision as well as night blindness. The liver can store about 95% of the body's reserves of Vitamin A. It is needed daily, and there are plenty of foods which contain it, so that the person on a diet can easily suit his special needs. Foods highest in Vitamin A, in the order of the Vitamin A content per average portion, are:

    Greens
    Carrots
    Liver
    Hubbard Squash
    Sweet Potatoes
    Cod Liver Oil
    Apricots Green
    Beans Peaches
    Tomato Juice
    Butter Peas

Prunes
Oleomargarine
Milk Cheese

Vitamin B Complex contains Thiamine or Bi, Riboflavin or B2, Niacin, Folic Acid and Para-aminobenzoic
Acid. There are several more B Complex substances that
are being discovered, but these will have to do for now.
Thiamine is invaluable for health and growth. Be sure
you get enough of it. You'll get your greatest amounts
of Thiamine in these foods, in the order named:

Pork
Dried Brewer's Yeast
Gluten Bread
Dried Beans and Peas
Whole Wheat or Enriched Bread
Corn Bread
Lamb
Peanuts
Milk
Oatmeal
Potatoes
Collards
Kale
Beef
Egg
Poultry and Fish
Asparagus
Brussels Sprouts

Riboflavin is necessary for health. It is good for the nerves, the digestion, the skin and the eyes. It helps keep you young—makes you look well. If your skin is too dry, if there are cracks in the corners of your mouth and your eyes are dull, you undoubtedly lack Riboflavin, and should add it to your diet. It is not easily destroyed in cooking, unless you add baking soda to your vegetables to keep them green. Baking soda will kill this valuable vitamin immediately I Riboflavin is found in the following good foods, in the order named:

Liver
Dried Brewer's Yeast
Milk
Prunes
Fish
Beef
Dried Beans and Peas
Pork
Green Beans
Eggs
Chicken
Spinach
Cheese
Peanuts
Cauliflower

Niacin is good for digestive troubles, for skin rash, and for sore tongue, and improves strength. Here are the best foods for Niacin, in the order in which this vitamin appears in the average serving:

Liver
Dried Brewer's Yeast
Pork
Bran
Salmon
Poultry
Beef
Peanuts
Gluten Bread
Whole Wheat and Enriched Bread
Potatoes
Carrots
Milk
Eggs

Vitamin C, or Ascorbic Acid, helps to cure infections and heal wounds rapidly. It is good for the teeth, for the gums, for the skin and for the general well-being. There are those who say it helps prevent grey hair, when taken with Calcium Pantothenate. Nothing definite has been proved about that, however. Foods containing Vitamin C should form a substantial part of your diet. In the order in which they contain this vitamin, they are:

Grapefruit
Strawberries
Oranges
Cantaloupe
Cabbage
Turnips

Sweet Potatoes
White Potatoes
Tomatoes
Avocados
Watermelons
Pineapples
Lettuce
Bananas
Peaches, Apples and Pears

Vitamin D, or the Sunshine Vitamin, helps build bones and teeth. It is developed mostly by sunlight, and even by the rays of sunlamps which have ultraviolet rays. It is also found in:

Oysters
Tuna Fish
Fish Liver

Vitamin P, or Citrin, is found in paprika, fruits, vegetables and lemon rind, and in orange juice and orange peel. It helps capillary resistance in people suffering from vitamin deficiency.

Vitamin E helps protect the alimentary tract and muscles, and adds a feeling of well-being. It is found in meats, milk, grains, vegetables and wheat germ.

Vitamin K was isolated from alfalfa in 1939, and has been used since then for various illnesses. It is valuable in helping the blood to clot properly. It is made, too, from fish oils. Man's exact requirement of Vitamin K is not known, but this vitamin will undoubtedly be found

to be valuable, once it has been thoroughly tested. It is
also found in leafy vegetables such as turnip greens and
carrot tops.

So that's that! A lot of these foods rank high on
your non-fattening list, too. When you spend your
money—and your calories—for food, don't pay attention just to caloric values. Check up on the vitamin content, too. In no other way will you be sure to get your
money's worth, and be properly nourished.

And while you're learning about vitamins, you might
add a bit to your knowledge of proteins, too, for your
high-protein diet. You're supposed to eat 70 grams of
protein a day, you know, so you might as well learn
about that now, too. The foods that contain proteins,
in the order of their protein content, based on an average serving, are as follows, marked to show how you
can get your necessary 70 grams per day most easily.
But you must avoid the more fattening foods while you
are dieting, even if they are high in protein, and add vegetables and fruits which are not on this list, as they are
valuable, too.

Meats	24 grams
Fowl	22 grams
Fish	22 grams
Cottage Cheese	20 grams
Milk	15 grams
Eggs (2)	15 grams
High-protein Bread (2 slices)	10 grams

High-protein Macaroni and Spaghetti	10 grams
Soy Beans	8 grams
Enriched White Bread (2 slices)	5 grams
Enriched Macaroni an Spaghetti	5 grams
Dried Beans and Peas	5 grams
Peanuts	5 grams
Cheese, such as Cheddar or Swiss	5 grams
Oysters	4 grams
Oatmeal	4 grams
Whole Wheat Cereals	3 grams
Gelatin (unsweetened)	3 grams

It's up to you to learn as much as you can about the foods you eat. That means thinking—thinking yourself thin! Choose foods for flavor, but choose them for protein, vitamins and minerals as well.

Minerals are as important as the other food elements in a well-rounded diet. And they will be included in your foods, if you choose your foods well. Some additional minerals may be needed, if your doctor finds your system is deficient in them, but with the natural foods you'll be getting now, you may not need extra minerals at all.

Many people who are inclined to be anemic need Iron in their blood. And overweight people are anemic more frequently than you think. It isn't always the skinny folks who have blood that lacks the proper quantity of red corpuscles. Iron, in tablet form, frequently prevents serious illness. And Iron is found in the following foods, in the order named:

Liver
Oysters
Dried Beans and Peas
Turnip Tops
Meat
Beet Greens
Gluten Bread
Enriched Bread
Chard
Kale
Spinach
Eggs
Whole Wheat Cereals
Potatoes
Oatmeal
Lettuce
Raisins

Calcium is one of our most valuable body minerals, and too often people disregard it. You won't get too much Calcium, unless your doctor warns you against it for some special defect in you. It is found in the following foods, as usual in the order in which they are listed, and for average portions:

Milk
Turnip Greens
Cheese
Collards
Kale
Broccoli

Gluten Bread
Hot Biscuits—a use for them at last!
Cauliflower
Beet Greens
Figs
Spinach
Beans
Cheese
Molasses

The Calcium in spinach and beet greens, alas, is in a form which is not easily assimilated by the body.

Copper is a valuable mineral, too, though the system needs very little of it. It is found in lean meats and green vegetables. Manganese is found in the foods that contain Iron—but it is found in adequate quantities in the well-balanced diet you'll be eating. Phosphorus and Magnesium are found in apples, string beans, beets, broccoli, cabbage, eggs, milk, gluten and whole wheat.

Sodium, Potassium, Chlorine, Iodine, Fluorine and Sulphur are other items to be found in the body—and needed in foods, too. There are even traces of other minerals in the body—Cobalt, Aluminum and Boron. These are all found in your well-balanced diet, so you don't have to do any thinking about them.

You needn't regard yourself as a walking corner drug-store. These elements are needed for your body— but you can get them painlessly by choosing wisely the foods for you.

I hope that this chapter has made you understand a

little more about foods and food content—and about yourself. For all of these elements make you what you are. Taken in adequate quantities, they will help you stay well and strong, and look well and young. If your food lacks them, you'll become listless, your eyes and skin will be dull, and you'll look your age or older.

Meat, milk, eggs, fruits and green vegetables, properly chosen, will give you an interesting diet and provide you with the right proteins, vitamins and minerals. When your food is lacking in essential vitamins and minerals, or if you need more than the average amount because you've allowed your system to get run down, your doctor can easily prescribe inexpensive supplements.

So please study your vitamin and mineral lists. Learn them so well that you'll put them automatically in your diet in the right amounts. Remember that, on these lists, the first items contain large amounts, and the vitamin and mineral and protein content dwindles rapidly as you go down the list.

Ready to learn more about foods?

CHAPTER 14

Choose your weapons

THIS IS THE LAST DIFFICULT CHAPTER. After this, it's easy as pie, but not as fattening, to follow the regime for thinking yourself thin. But this is going to be hard work. You've got to study! Just as if you were back in school, or taking a special course. Fine discipline. So you may as well face it. And think of all you'll learn! I hope so, anyhow. After this, you can sit back leisurely and feel wise and comfortable while you're reading about getting back into shape. You can even begin to be a bit smug, if that will help.

Your mental attitude, combined with the right food and the right exercise, is the thing that will make you thin. It is also the thing that will make you feel better, and look—and actually be—younger, in every way but chronologically. We can't do much about the actual calendar, I'm afraid.

Outside of your mental attitude—which I've been emphasizing, and which I will keep on emphasizing, food is the most important thing to think about, now. Food makes you what you are. Food makes fat. The right kind of food also makes good skin, clear eyes, healthy hair, a robust constitution. Wouldn't you think, when food is that important, that everyone would try to learn a lot about it.

For example, which is more fattening, a potato or an apple? I bet you think it's a potato—unless you've already gone into the subject. Well, they're about equal! Each has about a hundred calories. And how does a doughnut rank? Well, that's over twice as fattening as either one. And what about tomato juice? Do you know that, except for slight vitamin differences, it's just as good as orange juice—and in some ways even better— lower in calories, high in vitamins?

A lot of folks think fruit isn't fattening—you've learned better than that and this chapter will confirm your knowledge. Still others believe that if they eat a green salad, simply covered with rich dressing, they are performing a wonderful diet deed—when they're actually eating a fattening dish.

Other people believe that yogurt isn't fattening—and has wonderful health-giving properties. So they eat large amounts of it—and wonder why they don't lose weight. Yogurt is a very good food. It's just as fattening as whole milk—that is, a half pint of it (eight ounces) has a caloric value of 165 calories, the caloric value of an equal amount of whole milk, whereas skimmed milk, which has the same good properties, on the whole, has only 84 calories, and tomato juice only 50. But think of all of the good bacteria that yogurt contains I Haven't you been hearing about that for years? Yogurt is fermented milk. It came into use because people had no refrigeration. It was the only form of milk people could drink, without fear of contamination or illness. The intestines of all healthy people contain great numbers of friendly bacteria, maybe a hundred million or so. We don't need the few that yogurt could give us, but actually doesn't! According to the newest authorities, as quoted in a recent issue of *Today's Health,* published by the American Medical Association, the bacteria in yogurt are digested in the stomach, and very few reach the colon at all ! In yogurt you get lactic acid, a little alcohol and the good bacteria—which digest quickly. By all means, eat yogurt! It is good for you. As good as milk. If you like it, it should form a part of your diet—but don't expect wonders from it. Acidophilus milk, skimmed milk and yogurt are all excellent foods— complete foods. In fact, later on I'll give you a recipe for home-made yogurt, so you can make it with skimmed milk, thus reducing its caloric content. But it isn't a miracle food!

The same with the other so-called wonder foods. They are all good. But they aren't any more wonderful than a lot of other things that you can eat. Wheat germ is excellent—and high in calories. Black strap molasses contains some minerals—and is high in carbohydrates and calories.

But you should be able to tell about foods for yourself. Why take other people's word? That's why I told you that you'd have to study. For I'm giving you the complete Tables of Food Composition, in terms of eleven nutrients, prepared by the Bureau of Human Nutrition and Home Economics, U.S. Department of Agriculture, in co-operation with the National Research Council.

These new Tables of Food Composition are included in few books, mostly intended for the medical profession. As far as I can discover they have never been reprinted for the layman—for the man or woman who wants to get thin but isn't supposed to understand enough about foods to form his own opinion.

All of the books on diet for the nonprofessional reader that I have been able to find take it for granted that the reader shouldn't know too much. The foods that are listed are given by their caloric value only, so the reader can't tell if these foods are high or low in protein or starch or fat, or how they rank when it comes to vitamins and minerals. I've tried to show you how important these elements are—they are just as important as the actual caloric value of food. You cannot judge foods by calories alone!

"Restored" cereals are not included, because no definite standards have been established for them. You won't be eating too many breads or cereals, I trust, except special high-protein products, but, of course, you'll be getting better values, if you buy those with added vitamins.

Frozen foods are not included, but you can take it for granted that frozen vegetables and meats are just about the same in content as fresh foods. It used to be thought that foods lost vitamins during freezing. Now experts say that, when foods are frozen as soon as possible, they lose no more than in the ordinary marketing of fresh foods. Frozen fruits usually have added sugar. Look out for those, and count the added sugar calories.

The other day a successful woman said to me, with the certainty that only a successful woman can assume, "When I have to reduce, I go on a pure-protein diet." I asked her if she didn't mean high-protein. "Oh, no, I mean pure-protein," she told me. "Just eggs and meat." Look at your tables! You'll see that there is no such thing as a "pure-protein" diet. You can choose your own high-protein foods that you like and need, and you won't be fooling yourself with false ideas.

So study your tables. Learn not only the actual contents of foods, but why certain foods are good for you. A study of these tables will be far better for you than any so-called food expose. You'll turn from a novice into an expert as you study them.

You needn't memorize these tables. Almost unconsciously, as you study them, you'll learn and remember quite a lot. The more you learn, the better off you'll be. Of course, you can always turn back to them for reference! But think how wise you'll feel when you know, without constant leafing of the pages. For example, I know that there are approximately 23 grams of protein in a three-ounce, 400-calorie portion of cheese—so one ounce gives me only 100 calories and more than ten grams of protein, and, with a cracker or two, forms a nutritious dessert or midnight snack. But I know of a

lot of other things that will give me just as much protein and which I might prefer. I get pleasure—and results—from these tables.

So—here they are. Your food tables. The basis of
your food knowledge, that will help you think yourself
thin. You can accept all of the information given here for
you as the most comprehensive that can be obtained.
These tables have been corrected up to this year.

MILK AND MILK PRODUCTS:

Food and approximate measure or common weight	Water	Food energy	Protein	Fat	Carbohydrate	Calcium	Iron	Vitamin A value	Thiamine	Riboflavin value	Niacin value	Ascorbic acid
Buttermilk, from skim milk, 1 cup	90	85	9	Tr.	12	288	0.2	10	0.09	0.43	0.3	3
Milk, cow:												
Fluid, whole, 1 cup	87	165	9	10	12	288	.2	390	.09	.42	.3	3
Fluid, nonfat (skim), 1 cup	90	85	9	Tr.	13	303	.2	10	.09	.44	.3	3
Evaporated (undiluted), 1 cup	74	345	18	20	25	612	.4	1,010	.12	.91	.5	3
Condensed (undiluted), 1 cup	27	980	25	26	168	835	.6	1,300	.16	1.19	.6	3
Dry, whole, 1 tablespoon	4	40	2	2	3	76	0	110	.02	.12	.1	1
Dry, nonfat solids, 1 tablespoon	4	30	3	Tr.	4	98	0	Tr.	.03	.15	.1	1
Milk, goat, fluid, 1 cup	87	165	8	10	11	315	.2	390	.10	.26	.7	2
Cheese, 1 ounce:												
Cheddar (1 in. cube)	37	115	7	9	1	206	.3	400	.01	.12	0	
Cheddar, processed	40	105	7	8	1	191	.3	370	Tr.	.12	0	
Cheese foods, Cheddar	43	90	6	7	2	162	.2	300	.01	.16	0	
Cottage, from skim milk	76	25	6	Tr.	1	27	.1	10	.01	.09	0	
Cream	51	105	3	10	1	19	1	410	Tr.	.06	Tr.	0
Swiss	39	105	8	8	Tr.	262	.3	410	Tr.	.11	Tr.	0
Cream, 1 tablespoon:												
Light	72	30	Tr.	3	1	15	0	120	Tr.	.02	Tr.	Tr.
Heavy	59	50	Tr.	5	Tr.	12	0	220	Tr.	.02	Tr.	Tr.
Beverages, 1 cup:												
Chocolate (all milk)	80	240	8	12	26	260	.5	350	.08	.40	.3	2
Cocoa (all milk)	79	235	10	12	27	298	1.0	400	.10	.46	.5	3
Chocolate flavored milk	83	185	8	6	26	272	.2	230	.08	.40	.2	2
Malted Milk	78	280	12	12	32	364	.8	680	.18	.56	—	3

Food and approximate measure or common weight	Water	Food energy	Protein	Fat	Carbohydrate	Calcium	Iron	Vitamin A value	Thiamine	Riboflavin	Niacin value	Ascorbic acid
MILK AND MILK PRODUCTS—*Continued*												
Desserts:												
Blanc mange, 1 cup	76	275	9	10	39	290	.2	390	.08	.40	.2	2
Custard, baked, 1 cup	77	285	13	13	28	283	1.2	840	.11	.49	.2	1
Custard pudding, canned, strained (infant food), 1 ounce	75	30	1	1	5	26	.1	60	Tr.	.04	Tr.	Tr.
Ice cream, plain:												
1/7 of quart brick	62	165	3	10	17	100	.1	420	.03	.15	.1	1
8 fluid ounces	62	295	6	18	29	175	.1	740	.06	.27	.1	1
FATS, OILS, RELATED PRODUCTS:												
Bacon, medium fat, broiled or fried, 2 slices.	13	95	4	9	Tr.	4	.5	0	.08	.05	.8	0
Butter, 1 tablespoon	16	100	Tr.	11	Tr.	3	0	460	Tr.	Tr.	Tr.	0
Fats, cooking (vegetable fats):												
1 cup	0	1,770	0	200	0	0	0	0	0	0	0	0
1 tablespoon	0	110	0	12	0	0	0	0	0	0	0	0
Lard 1 tablespoon	0	125	0	14	0	0	0	0	0	0	0	0
Margarine, 1 tablespoon	16	100	Tr.	11	Tr.	3	0	460	0	0	0	0
Oils, salad or cooking, 1 tablespoon	0	125	0	14	0	0	0	0	0	0	0	0
Salads dressings 1 tablespoon:												
French	406	0	Tr.	.5	3	0	0	0	0	0	0	0
Home-cooked	68	30	1	2	3	15	.1	80	.01	.03	Tr.	Tr.
Mayonnaise	16	90	Tr.	10	Tr.	2	.1	30	Tr.	Tr.	0	0

Food and approximate measure or common weight	Water	Food energy	Pro-tein	Fat	Carbo-hydrate	Cal-cium	Iron	Vitamin A value	Thia-mine	Ribo-flavin	Niacin value	Ascor-bic acid
EGGS:												
Eggs, raw, medium:												
1 whole	74	75	6	6	Tr.	26	1.3	550	.05	.14	Tr.	0
1 white	88	15	3	0	Tr.	2	.1	0	0	.08	Tr.	0
1 yolk	49	60	3	5	Tr.	25	1.2	550	.05	.06	Tr.	0
Eggs, dried, whole, 1 cup	5	640	51	45	3	205	9.5	4,040	.36	1.14	.3	0
MEAT, POULTRY, FISH:												
Beef, 3 ounces, without bone, cooked:												
Chuck	51	265	22	19	0	9	2.6	0	.04	.17	3.2	0
Hamburger	47	315	19	26	0	8	2.4	0	.07	.16	4.1	0
Sirloin	54	255	20	19	0	9	2.5	0	.06	.16	4.1	0
Beef, canned:												
Corned beef, medium fat, 3 ounces:	59	180	22	10	9	17	3.7	Q	.01	.20	2.9	0
Corned beef hash, 3 ounces	70	120	12	5	6	22	1.1	Tr.	.02	.11	2.4	0
Strained (infant food), 1 ounce	78	30	5	1	0	3	1.2	0	Tr.	.06	.9	0
Beef, dried, 2 ounces	48	115	19	4	0	11	2.9	0	0.4	.18	2.2	0
Beef and vegetable stew, 1 cup	79	250	13	19	17	31	2.6	2,520	.12	.15	3.4	15
Chicken, canned, boned, 3 ounces	62	170	25	7	0	12	1.5	0	.03	.14	5.4	0
Chile con came, canned (without beans), 1/3 cup	67	170	0	13	5	32	1.2	130	.01	.10	1.9	—
Clams, raw, meat only, 4 ounces	80	90	15	2	4	109	7.9	120	.11	.20	1.8	—
Cod, dried, 1 ounce	12	105	23	1	0	14	1.0	0	.02	.13	3.1	0
Crab meat, canned or cooked, 3 ounces	77	90	14	2	0	38	.8	—	.04	.05	2.1	
Flounder, raw, 4 ounces	83	80	17	1	0	69	.9	—	.07	.06	1.9	—

Food and approximate measure or common weight	Water	Food energy	Pro-tein	Fat	Carbo-hydrate	Cal-cium	Iron	Vitamin A value	Thia-mine	Ribo-flavin	Niacin value	Ascor-bic acid
MEAT, POULTRY, FISH—Continued												
Haddock, fried, 1 fillet (4 by 3 by J4 in.)	67	160	19	6	7	18	.6	—	.04	.09	2.6	—
Halibut, broiled, 1 steak (4 by 3 by ½ in.)	64	230	33	10	0	18	1.0	—	.08	.09	13.1	—
Heart, beef, raw, 3 ounces	78	90	14	3	1	8	3.9	30	.50	.75	6.6	5
Kidneys, beef, raw, 3 ounces	75	120	13	7	1	S	6.7	980	.32	2.16	5.5	11
Lamb, leg roast, cooked, 3 ounces	56	230	20	16	0	9	2.6	0	.12	.21	4.4	0
Lamb, canned, strained (infant food), 1 ounce	79	30	4	1	0	5	7	0	.01.	07	1.1	0
Liver, beef, fried, 2 ounces	57	120	13	4	5	5	4.4	30,330	.15	2.25	8.4	18
Liver, canned, strained (infant food), 1 ounce	78	30	5	1	Tr.	7	2.0	5-440	.01	.61	1.8	—
Mackerel, canned, solids and liquid, 3 ounces	66	155	16	9	0	157	1.8	370	.05	.18	4.9	—
Oysters, meat only, raw, 1 cup (13-19 medium size oysters, selects)	80	200	24	5	13	226	13.4	770	.35	.48	2.8	—
Oyster stew, 1 cup with 6 to 8 oysters	80	245	17	13	14	262	7.0	820	.21	.46	1.6	—
Pork loin or chops, cooked, 3 ounces without bone	50	285	20	22	0	9	2.6	0	.71	.20	4.3	0
Pork, cured ham, cooked, 3 ounces without bone	39	140	20	2S	Tr.	9	1.5	0	.46	.18	3.5	0

MEAT, POULTRY, FISH—Continued

Food and approximate measure or common weight	Water	Food energy	Protein	Fat	Carbohydrate	Calcium	Iron	Vitamin A value	Thiamine	Riboflavin	Niacin value	Ascorbic acid
Pork luncheon meat, canned, spiced, 2 ounces	55	165	8	14	1	5	1.2	0	18	.12	1.6	0
Salmon, canned, pink, 3 ounces	70	120	17	5	0	159	.7	60	.03	.16	6.8	0
Sardines, canned in oil, drained solids, 3 ounces	57	180	22	9	1	328	2.3	190	.01	.15	4.1	0
Sausage:												
Bologna, 1 piece (1 by 1½ in. diam.)	62	465	31	34	8	19	4.6	0	.37	.40	5.7	0
Frankfurter, 1 cooked	62	90	17	Tr.	4	29	2.0	0	.05	.11	1.6	—
Shad, raw, 4 ounces	70	190	21	11	0	—	.6	—	.17	.27	9.6	—
Shrimp, canned, meat only, 3 ounces	66	110	23	1	—	98	2.6	50	.01	.03	1.9	0
Soups, canned, ready-to-serve:												
Beef, 1 cup	91	100	6	4	11	15	.5	—	—	.12	—	—
Chicken, 1 cup	94	75	4	2	10	20	.5	—	.02	—	1.5	—
Chicken, strained (infant food), 1 ounce	87	15	1	1	2	11	.1	70	Tr.	.03	.1	Tr.
Clam chowder, 1 cup	91	85	5	2	12	36	3.6	—	—	—	—	—
Tongue, beef, raw, 4 ounces	68	235	19	17	Tr.	10	3.2	0	.14	.33	5.7	0
Tuna fish, drained solids, 3 ounces	60	170	25	7	0	7	1.2	70	.04	.10	10.9	0
Veal cutlet, cooked, 3 ounces without bone	60	185	24	9	0	10	3.0	0	.07	.24	5.2	0

Food and approximate measure or common weight	Water	Food energy	Pro-tein	Fat	Carbo-hydrate	Cal-cium	Iron	Vitamin A value	Thia-mine	Ribo-flavin	Niacin value	Ascor-bic acid
MATURE BEANS AND PEAS; NUTS:												
Almonds, shelled, unblanched, 1 cup	5	850	26	77	28	361	6.2	0	.35	.95	6.5	Tr.
Beans, canned or cooked, 1 cup:												
Red kidney	76	230	15	1	42	102	4.9	0	.12	.12	2.0	0
Navy or other varieties with:												
Pork and tomato sauce	71	295	15	5	48	107	4.7	220	.13	.09	1.2	7
Pork and molasses	70	325	15	8	50	146	5.5	90	.13	.09	1.2	7
Beans, lima, dry, 1 cup	13	610	38	2	113	124	13.7	0	.88	.32	3.6	3
Brazil nuts, shelled, 1 cup	5	905	20	92	15	260	4.8	Tr.	1.21	—	—	—
Coconut, dried, shredded (sweetened), 1 cup	3	345	2	24	33	27	2.2	0	Tr.	Tr.	Tr.	0
Cowpeas, dry, 1 cup	11	685	46	3	123	154	13.0	60	1.84	.32	4.5	3
Peanuts, roasted, shelled, 1 cup	3	805	39	64	34	107	2.7	0	.42	.19	23.3	0
Peanut butter, 1 tablespoon	2	90	4	8	3	12	.3	0	.02	.02	2.6	0
Peas, split, dry, 1 cup	10	690	49	2	123	66	10.2	740	1.53	.56	6.3	4
Pecans, 1 cup halves	3	750	10	79	14	80	2.6	50	.77	.12	1.0	2
Soybeans, dry, 1 cup	7	695	73	38	73	477	16.8	230	2.25	.65	4.9	Tr.
Walnuts, English, 1 cup halves	3	655	15	64	16	83	2.1	30	.48	.13	1.2	3
VEGETABLES:												
Asparagus:												
Cooked, 1 cup cut spears	92	35	4	Tr.	6	33	1.8	1,820	.23	.30	2.1	40
Canned green, 6 spears, medium size	92	20	2	Tr.	3	18	1.8	770	.06	.08	.9	17
Canned bleached, 6 spears, medium size	92	20	2	Tr.	3		1.0	70	.05	.07	.8	17

Food and approximate measure or common weight	Water	Food energy	Protein	Fat	Carbohydrate	Calcium	Iron	Vitamin A value	Thiamine	Riboflavin	Niacin value	Ascorbic acid
VEGETABLES —Continued												
Beans, lima, immature, cooked, 1 cup	7 5	150	8	1	29	46	2.7	460	.22	.14	1.8	24
Beans, snap, green, cooked, 1 cup	92	25	2	Tr.	6	45	.9	830	.09	.12	.6	18
Beets, cooked, diced, 1 cup	88	70	2	Tr.	16	35	1.2	30	.03	.07	.5	11
Broccoli, cooked, flower, 1 cup	90	45	5	Tr.	8	195	2.0	5,100	.10	.22	1.2	111
Brussels, sprouts, cooked, 1 cup	85	60	6	1	12	44	1.7	520	.05	.16	.6	61
Cabbage, 1 cup:												
Raw, shredded	92	25	1	Tr.	5	46	.5	80	.06	.05	.3	50
Cooked	92	40	2	Tr.	9	78	.8	150	.08	.08	.5	53
Carrots:												
Raw, grated, 1 cup	88	45	1	Tr.	10	43	.9	13,200	.06	.06	.7	7
Cooked, diced, 1 cup	91	45	1	1	9	38	.9	18,130	.07	.07	.7	6
Canned, strained (infant food), 1 ounce	92	10	Tr.	0	2	7	.2	2,530	.01	.01	.1	1
Cauliflower, cooked, flower buds, 1 cup	92	30	3	Tr.	6	26	1.3	110	.07	.10	.6	34
Celery, 1 cup:												
Raw, diced	94	20	1	Tr.	4	50	.5	0	.05	.04	.4	7
Cooked diced, 1 cup	91	45	1	1	5	65	.6	0	.05	.04	.4	6
Collards, cooked, 1 cup	87	75	7	1	14	473	3.0	14,500	.15	.46	3.2	84
Corn, sweet:												
Cooked, 1 ear (5 in. long)	75	85	3	1	20	5	.6	390	.11	.10	1.4	8
Canned, solids and liquid, 1 cup	80	170	5	1	41	10	1.3	520	.07	.13	2.4	14
Cowpeas, immature seed, cooked, 1 cup	75	150	11	1	25	59	4.0	620	.46	.13	1.3	32
Cucumbers, raw, 6 slices, ½ in. thick, center section)	96	5	Tr.	0	1	5	.2	0	.02	.02	.1	4
Dandelion greens, cooked, 1 cup	86	80	5	1	16	337	5.6	27,310	.23	.22	1.3	29

VEGETABLES—*Continued*

Food and approximate measure or common weight	Water	Food energy	Pro-tein	Fat	Carbo-hydrate	Cal-cium	Iron	Vitamin A value	Thia-mine	Ribo-flavin	Niacin value	Ascor-bic acid
Endive, raw, 1 pound -	93	90	7	1	18	359	7.7	13,600	.30	.53	1.8	49
Kale, cooked, 1 cup	87	45	4	1	8	248	2.4	9,220	.08	.25	1.9	56
Lettuce, headed, raw, 2 large or 4 small leaves	95	5	1	Tr.	1	11	.2	270	.02	.04	.1	4
Mushrooms, canned, solids and liquid, 1 cup	93	30	3	Tr.	9	17	2.0	0	.04	.60	4.8	—
Mustard greens, cooked, 1 cup	92	30	3	Tr.	6	308	4.1	10,050	.08	.25	1.0	63
Okra, cooked, 8 pods (3 in. long, 5/8 in. diam.)	90	30	2	Tr.	6	70	.6	630	.05	.05	.7	17
Onions, raw:												
Mature (1 onion 2½ in. diam.) ,,	88	50	2	Tr.	11	35	.6	60	.04	.04	.2	10
Young green, 6 small onions without tops	88	25	Tr.	Tr.	5	68	.4	30	.02	.02	.1	12
Parsnips, cooked, 1 cup	84	95	2	1	22	88	1.1	0	.09	.16	.3	19
Peas, green:												
Cooked, 1 cup	82	110	8	1	19	35	3.0	1,150	.40	.22	3.7	24
Canned, strained (infant food), 1 ounce	87	15	1	Tr.	2	5	.4	180	.03	.02	.3	2
Peppers, green, raw, 1 medium	92	15	1	Tr.	4	7	.3	400	.02	.04	.2	77
Potatoes:												
Baked, 1 medium(2½in.diam.)	74	95	2	Tr.	22	13	.8	20	.11	.05	1.4	17
Boiled in skin, 1 medium (2½ in. diam.)	78	120	3	Tr.	27	16	1.0	30	.14	.06	1.6	22

VEGETABLES—Continued
Potatoes: (continued)

Food and approximate measure or common weight	Water	Food energy	Pro-tein	Fat	Carbo-hydrate	Cal-cium	Iron	Vitamin A value	Thia-mine	Ribo-flavin	Niacin value	Ascor-bic acid
Boiled after peeling, 1 medium (2½ in. diam.)	78	105	3	Tr.	24	14	.9	20	.12	.04	1.3	17
French-fried, 8 pieces (2 by ½ by ½ in.)	20	155	2	8	21	12	.8	20	.07	.04	1.3	11
Potato chips, 10 medium (2 in. diam.)	3	110	1	7	10	6	.4	10	.04	.02	.6	2
Pumpkin, canned, 1 cup	90	75	2	1	18	46	1.6	7,750	.04	.14	1.2	—
Radishes, raw, 4 small	94	5	Tr.	0	1	7	.2	10	.01	Tr.	.1	5
Rutabagas, cooked, cubed or sliced, 1 cup	91	50	1	Tr.	12	85	.6	540	.08	.11	1.1	33
Sauerkraut, canned, drained solids, 1 cup	91	30	2	Tr.	7	54	.8	60	.05	.10	.2	24
Soybean sprouts, raw, 1 cup	86	50	7	1	6	51	1.1	190	.24	.21	.9	14
Spinach:												
Cooked, 1 cup	91	45	6	1	6	223	3.6	21,200	.14	.36	1.1	54
Canned, strained (infant food), 1 ounce	94	5	1	Tr.	1	22	.4	1,190	.01	.03	.1	2
Squash												
Summer, cooked, diced, 1 cup	95	35	1	Tr.	8	32	.8	550	.08	.15	1.3	23
Winter, baked, mashed, 1 cup	86	95	4	1	23	49	1.6	12,690	.10	.31	1.2	14
Winter, canned, strained (infant food), 1 ounce	91	10	Tr.	Tr.	2	9	.1	560	.01	.02	.1	1
Sweetpotatoes, peeled, 1 sweetpotato:												
Baked (5 by 2 in.)	61	185	3	1	41	44	1.1	11,410	.12	.08	.9	28
Boiled (5 by 2½ in.)	69	250	4	1	57	62	1.4	15,780	.18	.11	1.3	41

Food and approximate measure or common weight	Water	Food energy	Protein	Fat	Carbohydrate	Calcium	Iron	Vitamin A value	Thiamine	Riboflavin	Niacin value	Ascorbic acid
VEGETABLES—Continued												
Tomatoes:												
Raw, 1 medium (2 by 2½ in.) —	94	30	2	Tr.	6	16	.9	1,640	.08	.06	.8	35
Canned or cooked, 1 cup	94	45	2	Tr.	9	17	1.5	2,540	.14	.08	1.7	40
Tomato juice, canned, 1 cup	94	50	2	Tr.	10	17	1.0	2,540	.12	.07	1.8	38
Turnips, cooked, diced, 1 cup	92	40	1	Tr.	9	62	.8	Tr.	.06	.09	.6	28
Turnip greens, cooked, 1 cup	90	45	4	1	8	376	3.5	15,370	.09	.59	1.0	87
Vegetables, mixed, canned, strained (infant food), 1 ounce	90	10	Tr.	0	2	9	.3	—	.01	.01	.1	1
FRUITS:												
Apples, raw, 1 medium (2½ in. diam.)	84	75	Tr.	1	20	8	.4	120	.05	.04	.2	6
Applejuice, fresh or canned, 1cup	86	125	Tr.	0	34	15	1.2	90	.05	.07	Tr.	2
Apple betty, 1 cup	64	345	4	7	70	34	.2	370	.13	.09	1.1	3
Applesauce, canned, sweetened, 1 cup	80	185	1	Tr.	59	10	1.0	80	.05	.03	.1	3
Apricots:												
Raw, 3 apricots	85	55	1	Tr.	14	17	.5	2,990	.03	.05	.9	7
Canned in syrup, 4 medium halves and 2 tablespoons syrup	77	95	1	Tr.	26	12	.4	1,650	.02	.03	.4	5
Canned, strained (infant food), 1 ounce	83	15	Tr.	Tr.	4	6	.3	480	.01	.01	.1	1
Dried, cooked, unsweetened, fruit and liquid, 1 cup	75	240	5	Tr.	62	80	4.6	6,900	.01	.14	2.8	9
Avocados, raw, ½ peeled fruit 3.5 by 3¼ in.)	65	280	2	30	6	11	.7	330	.07	.15	1.3	18

FRUITS-Continued

Food and approximate measure or common weight	Water	Food energy	Protein	Fat	Carbohydrate	Calcium	Iron	Vitamin A value	Thiamine	Riboflavin	Niacin	Ascorbic acid
Bananas, raw, 1 medium (6 by 1½ in.)	75	90	1	Tr.	23	8	.6	430	.04	.05	.7	10
Blackberries, raw, 1 cup	85	80	2	1	18	46	1.3	280	.05	.06	.5	30
Blueberries, raw, 1 cup	83	85	1	1	21	22	1.1	400	.04	.03	.4	23
Cantaloups, raw, ½ melon (5 in. diam.)	94	35	1	Tr.	8	31	.7	6,190	.09	.07	.9	59
Cherries, 1 cup pitted:												
Raw	83	65	1	1	16	19	.4	710	.05	.06	.4	9
Canned red sour	87	120	2	1	30	28	.8	1,840	.07	.04	.4	14
Cranberry sauce, sweetened, 1 cup	48	550	Tr.	1	142	22	.8	80	.06	.06	.3	5
Dates, "fresh" and dried, pitted and cut, 1 cup	20	505	4	1	134	128	3.7	100	.16	.17	3.9	0
Figs, raw, 3 small (1½ in. diam.)	78	90	2	Tr.	22	62	.7	90	.06	.06	.6	2
Figs, dried, 1 large (2 by 1 in.)	24	55	1	Tr.	14	39	.6	20	.03	.02	.4	0
Fruit cocktail, canned, solids and liquid, 1 cup	81	180	1	1	48	23	1.0	410	.03	.03	.9	5
Grapefruit, raw, 1 cup sections	89	75	1	Tr.	20	43	.4	20	.07	.04	.4	78
Grapefruit juice:												
Canned unsweetened, 1 cup	89	90	1	Tr.	24	20	.7	20	.07	.04	.4	85
Frozen concentrate, 6-ounce can	58	295	4	1	77	63	2.4	60	.24	.13	1.4	272
Grapes, 1 cup:												
Americantype(slipskin)	82	85	2	2	18	20	.7	90	.07	.05	.3	5
European type (adherent skin)	82	100	1	1	26	26	.9	120	.09	.06	.4	6
Grape juice, bottled, 1 cup	81	170	1	0	46	25	.8	—	.09	.12	.6	Tr.

FRUITS—Continued

Food and approximate measure or common weight	Water	Food energy	Protein	Fat	Carbohydrate	Calcium	Iron	Vitamin A value	Thiamine	Riboflavin	Niacin value	Ascorbic acid
Lemon juice, fresh, 1 cup	91	60	1	Tr.	19	34	.2	0	.11	.01	.3	122
Lime juice, fresh, 1 cup	91	60	1	0	20	34	.2	0	.11	.01	.3	65
Oranges, 1 medium (3 in. diam.)	87	70	1	Tr.	17	51	.6	290	.12	.04	.4	77
Orange juice:												
Fresh, 1 cup	88	110	2	Tr.	27	47	.5	460	.19	.06	.6	122
Canned, unsweetened, 1 cup	88	110	2	Tr.	27	25	.7	240	.17	.04	.6	103
Frozen concentrate, 6-ounce can	58	300	5	1	75	69	2.0	670	.48	.11	1.5	285
Papayas, raw, cubed, 1 cup	89	70	1	Tr.	18	36	.5	3,190	.06	.07	.5	102
Peaches:												
Raw, 1 medium (2 ½ by 2 in. diam.)	87	45	1	Tr.	12	8	.6	880	.02	.05	.9	1
Canned in syrup, solids and liquid, 1 cup	81	175	1	Tr.	47	13	1.0	1,160	.02	.05	1.8	11
Canned, strained (infant food), 1 ounce	83	15	Tr.	Tr.	4	2	.3	180	.01	.01	.2	1
Dried, cooked, unsweetened, 1 cup (10-12 halves and 6 tablespoons liquid)	76	225	2	1	59	38	5.9	2,750	.01	.16	4.3	11
Pears:												
Raw, 1 pear (3 by 2½ in. diam.)	83	95	1	1	24	20	.5	30	.03	.06	.2	6
Canned in syrup, 2 medium size halves and 2 tablespoons syrup	81	80	Tr.	Tr.	22	9	.2	Tr.	.01	.02	.2	2
Canned, strained (infant food), 1 ounce	86	15	Tr.	Tr.	4	3	.1	10	Tr.	.01	.1	Tr.

Food and approximate measure or common weight	Water	Food energy	Protein	Fat	Carbohydrate	Calcium	Iron	Vitamin A value	Thiamine	Riboflavin	Niacin value	Ascorbic acid
FRUITS—Continued												
Persimmons, Japanese, raw, seedless kind, 1 persimmon (2¼ in. diam.)	78	95	1	Tr.	24	7	.4	3,270	.06	.05	Tr.	13
Pineapple:												
Raw, diced, 1 cup	85	75	1	Tr.	19	22	.4	180	.12	.04	.3	33
Canned in syrup, 2 small or 1 large slice and 2 tablespoons juice	78	95	Tr.	Tr.	26	35	.7	100	.09	.02	.2	11
Pineapple juice, canned, 1 cup	86	120	1	Tr.	32	37	1.2	200	.13	.04	.4	22
Plums, raw, 1 plum (2 in. diam.)	86	30	Tr.	Tr.	7	10	.3	200	.04	.02	.3	3
Prunes, cooked, unsweetened, 1 cup (16-18 prunes and ¾ cup liquid)	65	310	3	1	82	62	4.5	3,210	.07	.20	2.0	2
Prune juice, canned, 1 cup	80	170	1	0	46	60	4.3	—	.07	.19	1.0	2
Raisins, dried, 1 cup	24	430	4	1	114	125	5.3	80	.24	.13	.8	Tr.
Raspberries, red, raw, 1 cup	84	70	1	Tr.	17	49	1.1	160	.03	.08	.4	29
Rhubarb, cooked with sugar, 1 cup	63	385	1	Tr.	98	112	1.1	70	.02	—	.2	17
Strawberries:												
Raw, 1 cup	90	55	1	1	12	42	1.2	90	.04	.10	.4	89
Frozen, 3 ounces	72	90	1	Tr.	23	19	.5	30	.02	.04	.2	55
Tangerines, 1 medium (2½ in. diam.)	87	35	1	Tr.	9	27	.3	340	.06	.02	.2	25
Tangerine juice, canned, 1 cup	89	95	2	1	23	47	.5	1,040	.15	.06	.6	64
Watermelon, ½ slice (¼ by 10 in.)	92	45	1	Tr.	11	11	.3	950	.08	.08	.3	10
GRAIN PRODUCTS:												
Barley, pearled, light, dry, 1 cup	11	710	17	2	160	32	4.1	0	.25	.17	6.3	0

GRAIN PRODUCTS—Continued

Food and approximate measure or common weight	Water	Food energy	Pro-tein	Fat	Carbo-hydrate	Cal-cium	Iron	Vitamin A value	Thia-mine	Ribo-flavin	Niacin value	Ascor-bic acid
Biscuit, baking powder, enriched flour, 1 biscuit (2 ½ in. diam.)	17	130	3	4	20	83	.7	0	.05	.08	.7	0
Bran flakes, 1 cup	4	115	4	1	32	24	2.0	0	.19	.09	3.5	0
Breads, 1 slice:												
Boston brown, unenriched	44	105	2	1	22	89	1.2	70	.04	.06	.7	0
Rye	35	55	2	Tr.	12	17	.4	0	.04	.02	.4	0
White, unenriched, 4 percent nonfat milk solids	35	65	2	1	12	18	.1	0	.01	.02	.2	0
White, enriched, 4 percent nonfat milk solids	35	65	2	1	12	18	.4	0	.06	.04	.5	0
White, enriched, 6 percent nonfat milk solids	34	65	2	1	12	21	.4	0	.06	.04	.5	0
Whole wheat	37	55	2	1	11	22	.5	0	.07	.03	.7	0
Cakes: Angel food, 2-inch sector (1/12 of cake, 8 in. diam.)	32	110	3	Tr.	23	2	.1	0	Tr.	.05	.1	0
Doughnuts, cake-type, 1 doughnut	19	135	2	7	17	23	.2	40	.05	.04	.4	0
Foundation, 1 square (3 by 2 by 1 ¼ in.)	25	230	4	8	36	82	.3	100	.02	.05	.2	0
Foundation, plain icing, 2-inch sector, layer cake (1/16 of cake 10 in diam.)	24	410	6	11	72	121	.5	150	.03	.08	.2	0
Fruit cake, dark, 1 piece (2 by 2 by ½ in.)	23	105	2	4	17	29	.8	50	.04	.04	.3	9

GRAIN PRODUCTS—*Continued*

Cakes: *(continued)*

Food and approximate measure or common weight	Water	Food energy	Pro- tein	Fat	Carbo- hydrate	Cal- cium	Iron	Vitamin A value	Thia- mine	Ribo- flavin	Niacin value	Ascor- bic acid
Gingerbread, 1 piece (2 by 2 by 2 in.)	30	180	2	7	28	63	1.4	50	.02	.05	.6	0
Plain cake and cupcakes, 1 cupcake (2¾, in. diam)	17	130	3	3	23	62	.2	50	.01	.03	.1	0
Sponge, 2-inch sector (1/12 of cake, 8 in. diam.)	32	115	3	2	22	11	.6	210	.02	.06	.1	0
Cereal foods, dry, precooked (infant food), 1 ounce	6	105	4	1	21	185	9.6	0	.34	.13	1.4	·
Cookies, plain and assorted, 1 3-inch cookie	5	110	2	3	19	6	.2	0	.01	.01	.1	0
Corn bread or muffins made with enriched, degermed corn meal, 1 muffin (2¾ in. diam.)	49	105	3	2	18	67	.9	60	.08	.11	.6	0
Corn flakes, 1 cup	4	95	2	Tr.	21	3	.3	0	.01	.02	.4	0
Corn grits, degermed, cooked, 1 cup:												
Unenriched	87	120	3	Tr.	27	2	.2	100	.04	.01	.4	0
Enriched	87	120	3	Tr.	27	2	.7	100	.11	.08	1.0	0
Crackers:												
Graham, 4 small or 2 medium	6	55	1	1	10	3	.3	0	.04	.02	.2	0
Soda, plain, 2 crackers (2½ in. diam.)	6	45	1	1	8	2	.1	0	.01	.01	.1	0
Farina, enriched, cooked, 1 cup	89	105	3	Tr.	22	7	.5	0	.10	.07	.4	0

Food and approximate measure or common weight	Water	Food energy	Protein	Fat	Carbohydrate	Calcium	Iron	Vitamin A value	Thiamine	Riboflavin	Niacin value	Ascorbic acid
GRAIN PRODUCTS—Continued												
Macaroni, cooked, 1 cup:												
Unenriched	61	210	7	1	42	13	.8	0	.03	.02	.7	0
Enriched	61	210	7	1	42	13	1.5	0	.24	.15	2.0	0
Muffins, made with enriched flour. 1 muffin (2 ¾ in. diam.)	37	135	4	4	20	99	.8	50	.09	.10	.7	0
Noodles, containing *egg*, unenriched, cooked, 1 cup	84	105	4	1	20	6	.6	60	.05	.03	.6	0
Oatmeal or rolled oats:												
Cooked, 1 cup	85	150	5	3	26	21	1.7	0	.22	.05	.4	0
Precooked (infant food), dry, 1 ounce	7	105	4	1	*19*	225	8.9	0	.36	.10	.7	0
Pancakes, baked, wheat, with enriched flour, 1 cake (4 in. diam.)	5 5	60	2	2	7	43	.4	50	.05	.06	.3	Tr.
Pies, 4-inch sector (9 in. diam.):												
Apple	48	330	3	13	53	9	.5	220	.04	.02	.3	1
Custard	59	265	7	11	34	162	1.6	290	.07	.21	.4	0
Lemon meringue	47	300	4	12	45	24	.6	210	.04	.10	.2	1
Mince	43	340	3	9	*61*	22	3.0	10	.09	.05	.5	1
Pumpkin	59	265	5	12	34	70	1.0	2,480	.04	.15	.4	0
Pretzels, 5 small sticks	8	20	Tr.	Tr.	. 4	1	0	0	Tr.	Tr.	Tr.	0
Rice, cooked, 1 cup:												
Converted	72	205	4	Tr.	45	14	.5	0	.10	.02	1.9	0
White or milled	71	200	4	Tr,	44	13	.5	0	.02	.01	.7	0
Rice, puffed, 1 cup	4	55	1	Tr.	12	3	.3	0	.01	.01	.1	0

Food and approximate measure or common weight	Water	Food energy	Protein	Fat	Carbohydrate	Calcium	Iron	Vitamin A value	Thiamine	Riboflavin	Niacin value	Ascorbic acid
GRAIN PRODUCTS—Continued												
Rolls, plain, enriched, 1 roll (12 per pound)	29	120	3	2	21	21	.7	0	.09	.06	.8	0
Spaghetti, unenriched, cooked, 1 cup	61	220	7	1	44	13	.9	0	.03	.02	.7	0
Waffles, baked, with enriched flour, 1 waffle (4½ by 5½ by ½ in.)	40	215	7	t	28	144	1.4	270	.14	.20	1.0	0
Wheat flours:												
Whole, 1 cup stirred	12	400	16	2	85	49	4.0	0	.66	.14	5.2	0
All purpose or family flour:												
Unenriched, 1 cup sifted	12	400	12	1	84	18	.9	0	.07	.05	1.0	0
Enriched, 1 cup sifted	12	400	12	1	84	18	3.2	0	.48	.29	3.8	0
Wheat germ, 1 cup stirred	11	245	17	7	34	57	5.5	0	1.39	.54	3.1	0
Wheat, shredded, 1 large biscuit, 1 ounce.	6	100	3	1	23	13	1.0	0	.06	.03	1.3	0
SUGARS, SWEETS:												
Candy, 1 ounce:												
Caramels	7	120	1	3	22	36	.7	50	.01	.04	Tr.	Tr.
Chocolate, sweetened, milk	1	145	2	9	16	61	.6	40	.03	.11	.2	0
Fudge, plain	5	115	Tr.	3	23	14	.1	60	Tr.	.02	Tr.	Tr.
Hard	1	110	0	0	28	0	0	0	0	0	0	0
Marshmallows	15	90	1	0	23	0	0	0	0	0	0	0
Chocolate syrup, 1 tablespoon	39	40	Tr.	Tr.	11	3	.3	—	—	—	—	—

Food and approximate measure or common weight	Water	Food energy	Pro-tein	Fat	Carbo-hydrate	Cal-cium	Iron	Vitamin A value	Thia-mine	Ribo-flavin	Niacin value	Ascor-bic acid
SUGAR, SWEETS—*Continued*												
Honey, strained or extracted, 1 tablespoon	20	60	Tr.	0	17	1	.2	0	Tr.	.01	Tr.	1
Jams, marmalades, preserves, 1 tablespoon	28	55	Tr.	Tr.	14	2	.1	Tr.	Tr.	Tr.	Tr.	1
Molasses, cane, 1 tablespoon:												
Light	24	50	—	—	13	33	.9	—	.01	.01	Tr.	—
Blackstrap	24	45	—	—	11	116	2.3	—	.02	.04	.3	—
Syrup, table blends, 1 tablespoon	25	55	O	O	15	9	.8	0	0	Tr.	Tr.	0
Sugar, 1 tablespoon:												
Granulated, cane or beet	Tr.	50	0	0	12	—	—	0	0	0	0	0
Brown	3	50	0	0	13	10	.4	0	0	0	0	0
MISCELLANEOUS:												
Beverages, carbonated, kola type, 1 cup	88	105	—	—	28	—	—	—	—	—	—	—
Bouillon cubes, 1 cube	5	2	Tr.	Tr.	0	—	—	—	—	.07	1.0	0
Chocolate, unsweetened, 1 ounce	2	140	2	15	8	28	1.2	20	.01	.06	.3	9
Gelatin dessert, plain, ready-to-serve, 1 cup	83	155	4	0	36	0	0	0	0	0	0	0
Olives, pickled "mammoth" size, 10 olives:												
Green	75	70	1	7	2	48	.9	160	Tr.	—	—	—
Ripe, Mission variety	72	105	1	12	1	48	3	40	Tr.	Tr.	—	—

Food and approximate measure or common weight	Water	Food energy	Pro-tein	Fat	Carbo-hydrate	Cal-cium	Iron	Vitamin A value	Thia-mine	Ribo-flavin	Niacin value	Ascor-bic acid
MISCELLANEOUS—*Continued*												
Pickles: *continued*												
Pickles:												
Dill, cucumber, 1 large (4 in. long)	9J	15	1	Tr.	3	34	1.6	420	Tr.	.09	.1	8
Sweet, cucumber or mixed, 1 pickle (2 ¾ in. long)	70	20	Tr.	Tr.	5	3	.3	20	0	Tr.	Tr.	1
Sherbet, ½ cup	68	120	1	0	29	48	0	0	.02	.07	0	0
Vinegar, 1 tablespoon	—	2	0	—	1	1	.1	—	—	—	—	—
White sauce, medium, 1 cup	73	430	11	33	23	305	.3	1,350	.09	.41	.3	1
Yeast:												
Compressed, baker's, 1 ounce	71	25	3	Tr.	3	7	1.4	0	.13	.59	8.0	0
Dried brewer's, 1 tablespoon	7	20	3	Tr.	3	8	1.5	0	.78	.44	2.9	0

These tables are reprinted here through the courtesy of the Bureau of Human Nutrition, U. S. Department of Agriculture.

CHAPTER 15

Good bye to yesterday

YESTERDAY WAS FINE. At least it was for me, and I hope it was for you, too. But yesterday is gone! And there's nothing we can do about that. The only use we can have for yesterday is to use it, occasionally, for reminiscing with old friends, and to learn what we can from it. If we can't learn from yesterday, we haven't lived very wisely.

As far as losing weight is concerned, we're going to go back to yesterday, briefly, here—and then never refer to it again. Personally, I think it's a lot more pleasant to talk about today and tomorrow. More rewarding, too. Yesterday's pretty dead! And there should be enough things happening today, and about to happen tomorrow, to keep you occupied, so that backward glances are unnecessary.

But now we're going back. A couple of weeks, anyhow. When you started to read this—a couple of weeks ago, if you've gone according to schedule—I suggested that you read one chapter a day. I asked you then to write down, each evening, everything you'd eaten during the day. I hope you did exactly that. It's an important part of the Think And Grow Thin regime.

Now, I want you to take out those notes. These should be complete daily records of what you've eaten — supposedly your normal food consumption during those two weeks or longer.

Now, turn to your Food Tables, given in the previous chapter, and write down, after each item of food, exactly how many calories it contained, together with the approximate carbohydrate and protein content. A hard task? Not as hard as studying the Food Tables in the previous chapter.

I've looked over some of those lists. They've always surprised me—but not nearly as much as they surprised the eaters. One fat girl, who thought she ate like a bird, because she omitted breakfast and had only a sandwich for lunch, found she ate about three times more, in calorie content, than she needed—and didn't get nearly enough protein, in proportion.

One day's menus for her, I remember, included:

LUNCH

Sandwich—Bread, Butter, Cheese	400 calories
Milk Chocolate, about	200
Gingerbread, with Whipped Cream	400

1,000

AT COCKTAIL TIME
    Two Cocktails   260 calories
    Peanuts and Crackers, about   200
                                         _____
                                                        460

DINNER
    Cream of Tomato Soup   150
    Chicken Pie   400
    Corn, about   70
    Salad, with Dressing   200
    French Pastry   250
    Bread and Butter   200
    Coffee with Cream and Sugar   200
                                         _____
                                                      1,470
AT ELEVEN
    Welsh Rarebit, with Toast, about   500
    Two Highballs   300
                                         _____
                                                        800
                                         _____
TOTAL CALORIES   3,730

Another day's list consisted of a richer sandwich, with dressing and more bread—a triple decker—tea and cakes instead of cocktails at five; a veal chop, rich with breading and cheese, with spaghetti and rich sauce, and dessert—but no midnight meal. The result was about the same. The food intake was over 3,000 calories per day, and always consisted of badly chosen foods.

all eaten in restaurants and chosen haphazardly. This girl went without breakfast as her idea of dieting, bought her own lunches, usually consisting of a sandwich, a drink and a dessert, at drug store counters; was taken out to a restaurant for dinner, where she usually ordered a soup high in calories, a rich meat dish, several rich accompaniments, and a heavy dessert. She usually ate only one roll, with two pats of butter, had cocktails before dinner, and ate what she thought was a light meal at eleven. When she began to think herself thin and change her food habits, she ate a sensible breakfast, a carefully selected luncheon, had one cocktail before dinner, then a high-protein meal, and, if she ate late at night, limited her meal to a glass of milk or fruit juice, or one highball or an apple and a bit of cheese. Her weight dropped forty pounds, from 165 to 125, over a period of three months; she lost ten years in appearance, went from size 40 to size 14, and says she never felt better in her life and wouldn't think of going back to her old way of living.

"I don't believe it, now," she told me, "that I ever lived that way—without really one thought of what I was doing. I'd read a lot about dieting, but never quite got the idea."

A man who thought he was dieting was eating over 2,500 calories a day.

"I eat out so much," he said, "that I can't possibly diet. People would think I was peculiar. I'm a professional man—have to go out with clients."

His list showed that his chief difficulty was a lack

of knowledge of food—and of himself. When he was put on the proper track, he was able to select the right meals for him, lost weight immediately—and no one even knew he was dieting, unless he told them, or they noted the improvement in his appearance and demeanor. I could tell you of dozens of other cases—but they're all so much alike! Unless you've already learned a lot about food, your lists will be similar—meals chosen without thought, heavy in carbohydrates and fats, and containing two or three times as many calories as necessary.

Most of the people who made lists went without breakfast—or had only coffee and fruit juices, the coffee usually rich with cream and sugar. This meant that they used up calories without benefit to them, and by the time lunch came they were hungry and irritable. Their lunch was either a sandwich and drink, with dessert —the sandwich top heavy with bread and lacking protein, because of its meager filling; the dessert and drink too full of carbohydrates—or a regulation heavy lunch, with meat, potatoes, bread and butter, and dessert. The average person had a drink before dinner, usually with a few nibbles or appetizers, which they didn't need at all— they may have needed appetite depressors, but not appetite encouragers—a heavy dinner, with soup or other liquids, gravies, small meat portions, heavy dressings and sauces, and unnecessary desserts. Then, too, many of these same people, not realizing how much they were eating, had something to eat late at night, the "something" adding from two to five hundred unnecessary calories to an already overcrowded food ration.

Two people I spoke to ate reasonable and fairly well selected meals—and spoiled their records by in-between-meal nibbling. One was a woman who stayed at home, and who ate her way through the day. She tasted while she cooked. She nibbled at fruit, candy, cookies or nuts all day long. Not a lot at a time. Just a nibble here and there—about 1,000 extra calories. The second was a man who ate sweets. He ate at least two chocolate bars, with or without nuts, at 400 calories a bar, and a couple of hundred extra calories of sweets a day—all between meals. Another man I know ate well balanced meals—and before his orders arrived he ate bread and butter. Each piece of bread or each roll averaged over 100 calories; each pat of butter, fifty calories. He ate at least six pieces of bread a day, with the same number of pats of butter—almost 1,000 extra calories.

I could go on and on. . . . You get the idea! And I'm not at all sure that your record is going to be perfect. In fact, if it is, and you're overweight, something is wrong. I'm sure, though, that you'll find, when you go over your records, that you've been eating incorrectly, without knowing just what you were doing.

When your records are finished, show them to your doctor when you visit him. They will give him a better picture of you than anything you could tell him.

And study these records yourself, so you'll understand what is wrong with your own eating habits. I think you'll understand yourself better than you ever did before—better than you could in any other way.

Now that you have the record of your past—even though it is only for the past two weeks—you won't have to go back into the past any more. You can close the book. You realize that your dietary habits are wrong. You may even have discovered why they are wrong.

Of course, you want to correct your bad eating habits. For you must realize that only by correcting them can you correct your obesity—your oversized dimensions and your overweight. It is just as easy to establish good eating habits as it is bad ones, when you realize what good eating habits are.

But you must change more than your habits of eating. You must change your viewpoint—your thoughts. In other words—you get the idea—you must think yourself thin. And it isn't going to be difficult, now that you're learning what to do.

So, study those old records. Find your errors, and admit to yourself what they are. You know the stories in which the hero or heroine "comes to realize," and then turns over a new leaf. This is your chance to be your own hero, to "come to realize" how wrong you've been, and to start over again. You should be grateful to Fate for a chance to start over on a new path.

Remember that a habit is formed consciously by doing something over and over again. And that you can quit a bad habit by stopping the thing you don't want to do each time you think of it. Remember each habit

is stopped or started by single omissions, by single repetitions. Each time you stop doing a thing that is
wrong, you have made a definite step in breaking the
chain of habit. Each time you repeat a good deed, you
have made a link in the new habit. It's as easy as that!
Your appetites may seem to be deeply formed. Perhaps
they are. You'll be surprised how easily they yield to
reason—to your conscious efforts. But you can do a lot
more than that. You can actually think yourself thin.

CHAPTER 16

Start to
think yourself thin

YOUR HARD WORK IS OVER! NO more tables to learn! No more calories to estimate in old menus. I hope, by now, you understand the values of the various foods you'll find available. And about high-protein foods. And foods that are low in calories. And about vitamins and minerals. Well, your charts are there for you—when you need them for reference. We can go on from there.

I hope you're all ready to go on. And eager and serious about getting thin. And staying thin. Ready to attract all the good things in life that will be there for you when, physically and mentally, you are at your best.

You are going to think yourself thin. Right away. Starting this very minute. You have, by now, I hope, the proper mental background. Goodness knows I've tried!

You've heard, I know, in dozens of books and magazine articles and radio talks, about the subconscious. And how you can make your subconscious work for you and with you. I wish I had space here to give you a whole course on psychology—a sort of refresher course, for I'm sure that is all you need. I feel, though, if you under-

169

stand what I've already said so far, that what I can tell you here will be enough to help you think yourself thin.

You realize, I know, that the thinking mind is the conscious mind. The subconscious does not think, psychologists say, but remembers and does what it is told. It is powerful—supposedly far more powerful than our thinking, awake mind. It is supposed to be like the submerged part of a glacier—hundreds of feet under the water for every ten feet or so above the surface. The subconscious is there, working, whether we are awake or asleep. The subconscious has a remarkable memory—it is supposed to retain everything that has ever happened to us. So it is the subconscious that can help or hold us back in our fight to become our better selves.

We must make our subconscious work for us as we think ourselves thin. Only in that way can we become thin permanently and with the right results. Now, I don't mean that we can't get thin without the help of the subconscious—for of course we can. A person on a starvation diet or a depleted diet will lose weight, even if he doesn't want to lose weight, either consciously or subconsciously. People in concentration camps become thin because they didn't get enough to eat. Simple as that. But it was also because they were miserably unhappy, so, in a way, the subconscious did have something to do with it. Any diet too low for sustenance will make you thin. That is a physiological fact. You actually do not need the subconscious to get thin I We all know dozens of people who have lost weight on a too-low diet without help from the subconscious at all.

Though, at that, usually those diets were helped a bit by the subconscious. We thought or said, "These diets will reduce," so the subconscious received the knowledge —and benefited by it. But the subconscious probably didn't do enough of the work!

On the other hand, I don't believe that you can possibly reduce only by thought—by letting your subconscious take over, without help from diet and exercise. You're fat undoubtedly because your mind and body both helped make you fat. I've tried to show you that. So, only by combining mind and body in the most sensible and scientific way can you get thin easily and improve your health and appearance at the same time. And once you've reached your right weight, stay thin and well.

If you have any organic disease—any illness of any kind—you should consult you physician. I'm not a physician or a magician. I can't cure serious ills. I wish I could. But I can promise you that I can help you reduce your weight by thought, if you'll follow the thought by prescribed action. First, an understanding of what I'm trying to tell you. Second, a visit to your own physician for a thorough check-up, as outlined in Chapter 10. Third, a study of the food tables. Fourth, comparing your usual diet with the tables, to discover how your diet has been wrong. Fifth, an understanding of how your mind and body work together to help you grow thin and stay thin. Sixth, the finding of a right diet for you. Seventh, the finding of right exercises for you. Eighth, a survey, for you, of the whole situation concerning you and thinking yourself thin. Of course, on the side, I hope you'll learn a lot more. But these are the basic things that you must do, if you're to get and stay slender by thinking yourself thin. If you'll think it over, now, I know you'll realize how far you've gone, already.

Thinking yourself thin has been recognized by most diet experts, even if they've never exactly put it in that form. All books on reducing use some form of psychology—with their diet and exercise advice. Individuals, too, have found this the best method, even if they've stumbled upon it without realizing its value.

Denise Darcel, the spectacular-looking French star, said to me in her delightfully accented English," I made up my mind to get thin. I said, 'I will not be fat! I am not fat!' But I was fat. I weighed over 150. Too much for me. So I say, 'What would I do if I were not fat?' I say, 'Once I am thin, I will be sensible not to be fat again.' So I do that. I pretend I am already thin. I eat and drink in moderation—what I would eat and drink if I weigh the right amount. So—I begin to lose. And I keep on thinking how I would live once I got thin. And I live that way. Always. All the time. Now I weigh 115 —just right for me. And I will not let myself gain. I keep on thinking I am thin and must not gain a single pound."

Ed Weiner, one of New York's popular publicity directors and writers, told me practically the same thing.

"I was quite fat last year," he said. "But as soon as I began to think about getting thin, I got thin. Of course I dieted at the same time. But it was the mental thing that was important. When I thought about getting thin, unconsciously I put my thoughts to work, and discarded the things that had made me fat. I did a lot of exercises—the sort I'd do if I were slender. I ate the things that would keep me slender. And before long I was slender. It's all in the mind—well, most of it, anyhow."

Certainly, the beauty parlors have put this same thought into their courses. In one of New York's most exclusive reduction salons, the surroundings are luxurious—silken pads on which to exercise, perfumed cubicles, gay enamels and chintzes. And the girls who instruct in the exercises are all slender and young and lovely. You couldn't possibly eat the wrong things, with those girls as examples. Unconsciously, you get the idea that if you do what they tell you to do—in exercise and diet—you'll look like them. You may not achieve that! But you'll get along a lot faster than if the surroundings were drab and the girls not quite as well formed.

At Elizabeth Arden's and Helena Rubinstein's salons in New York, the psychological effect of the exercise, diet and make-up of their courses is quite as important as the actual physical help. Of course, their desire is to sell their expensive cosmetic preparations—but they give good psychological help as well. You're bound to improve if you take their courses and use their cosmetics, for not only do the exercises and diets have real value, but the cosmetics often help your skin—and certainly you are Improved in appearance by clever make-up. More than that, your morale is strengthened. You can't help but feel that all of the luxury and beauty that has been created as a background must be of some help—so it is of some help. The diet and cosmetics, reduced to simple lists, boxes and jars, couldn't do as much as a salon visit, with mechanical aids, massage and supervised exercise and make-up. You are charged as much for psychological help as for the actual contributions to your physical well-being—but usually what you get is worth what you pay. The DuBarry Course is excellent, too, with its exercise and diets. The Coty productions, though usually without the aid of exercise salons, give you what you pay for them.

The beauty expert, Manya Kahn, has issued a home course that is especially valuable to the reducer who wants complete guidance. For those who do not want to lose weight, but just want to look better, too. In loose-leaf form, complete with easel, it gives a fourteen-day program in full color, with lots of photographs and drawings, for exercise, diet and poise. Published by Greystone, it is a valuable addition to the library of the person who wants to lose weight.

Miss Ann Delafield has done a lot to make women beauty conscious. She has given sensible advice, mixed with glamour and atmosphere, as to diet, make-up and exercise to thousands of women.

I remember, one time, speaking to the head of a big cosmetic company about one of their creams—a most expensive cream—practically a production number in packing and promotion.

"Look," I said, trying to be practical, "I've got the chemical analysis on this cream. You know as well as

I do that very little substance can go into the body through the skin—and that little doesn't stay there under the surface of the skin, anyhow, but is immediately absorbed. Isn't the skin a tough covering which actually can't be penetrated very well by these substances?"

"Yes," said the cosmetics expert, "that is true. But we advertise it in such a way that it's within the law. The cream does oil the skin—and you know that is good. And some of the ingredients undoubtedly are absorbed, in a way.'[1]

"I know that cream oils the skin and is good for it. But any inexpensive cream could do that. You charge a huge price for this—I happen to know that the cream costs you just a little more than the packaging. The whole thing couldn't cost a dollar."

"There's the advertising!" the expert said.

"But even that couldn't cost a great deal!"

The woman smiled and grew dreamy eyed.

"I know," she said, "but it's our best product. You see, we charge a great deal—because we sell hope with every jar!"

There you are — psychology again. The psychology that makes every reduction salon successful.

Even your visits to your doctor are tinged with psychology—as they should be, I'm sure. His advice must be expert advice. His words must be magic words. Aren't doctors a little more than human? We still regard our physicians in much the way primitive man looked upon witch doctors. His remedies are not just a simple mixture of drugs to produce certain effects. They have the aura of the unreal. The little bottle of appetite de-pressors that he may give us contains magic pills for losing weight. His diet lists are full of special proper-ties. It's just as well that we believe this. It helps us gain goals that might otherwise be far more difficult of achievement.

The reduction parlors, the gymnasiums, the doctors offices all offer us definite physical things. And with these come a lot of mental stimuli. Psychological pick-ups.

You may need those. I advise a visit to a doctor be-cause your own doctor can help you physically and men-tally. More than that, he can check up on your actual physical condition—and you need that personal check-up if you're overweight. I'm not a physician—and I couldn't prescribe for you long-distance if I were. Even if you were right here, I couldn't do a dozen things for you that your own doctor can do, as routine work. All I can do is to help you learn about obesity—and tell you the best way, in my opinion, to overcome it—keep it away forever—and feel better and look better at the same time.

The visit to your doctor is a "must"—one of the things that I insist on if I am to promise you success in thinking yourself thin. The beauty parlors are up to you. You may need them. You may not. Certainly, you don't have to have a beauty parlor to help you, if you are strong enough mentally to do for yourself the things that a beauty parlor does for you.

You can take care of your own subconscious, if you put your mind to it. Sometimes you actually must talk aloud to your subconscious. And don't think that this is a childish or half-witted thing to do! Some of the most brilliant and successful people I know find that they get their best results by speaking aloud to their subconscious! Certainly, you must do this when you are in a room alone, or people will think you've lost your mind. But try it! It's free! And it may help you. It has helped a lot of people.

The first thing in the morning, after you're up and around and have weighed yourself and written for five minutes in your note book—if you're making that psychological test of your own ideas, your own subconscious, actually—stand up very straight, your hands at your side. And say aloud:

"I am not fat! I am thin! I have allowed fat to accumulate on my body, but it does not belong there. I am a thin, well-formed human being, and I shall do all in my power to stay that way—to regain the appearance that I know is mine."

Say that several times. After the first day, omit the first sentence—and after that never again use the word "not" to your subconscious. Never plant a negative thought in your subconscious mind! A negative thought is bad for the subconscious, no matter what the thought may be. Never give the subconscious any ideas about failure, unhappiness or ugliness. Only by thinking success can you become successful. Only by giving to the subconscious mind ideas of what you want to be can you become that way.

That may sound oversimplified to you—and in a way

it is. For certainly these thoughts on success must be followed by actions to make you successful. But the thoughts must come first, or the actions cannot follow.

Over 30 years ago, Emile Coué of Nantes, France, had what was, at that time, a novel idea. He suggested that you put thirty knots in a piece of string. And that, twice a day, at morning and at night, you take the string and repeat thirty times, once each time you fingered one of the knots, "Every day in every way I'm getting better and better." The idea worked beautifully for some people—and not at all for others. So Coué and his theory faded out of sight. Why? Well, for one reason, he had nothing to sell, so there wasn't any promotional work back of him. If he'd had something to sell, and had been given a big advertising build-up, his theory might still be around. For another reason, he offered no follow-up ideas. Now, saying "Every day in every way I'm getting better and better," is planting a very fine idea in the subconscious. But unless you go on from there, the idea fades into nothingness. If everyone said that simple sentence every day—and then followed up the remark by trying, conscientiously, actually to be better and better every day, M. Coué's idea might have continued its initial spectacular success. Today, after these thirty years, we might be a different and a better people!

I'm not trying to reform the human race. Goodness knows, there seems to be enough room for reform, but I'm afraid my tiny candle would be extinguished by the first breeze. What I'm trying to do is to make those who read this feel and look better, by helping them grow more fit and slender. If I can do that, I shall give a great sigh of relief, and a prayer of happiness. I mean it. I'm serious about this. And I hope you are.

So let's get back to you and your subconscious—to that morning admonition. Speak to your subconscious—aloud if you like the idea. Use your own words—something like this:

"I am slender, actually. I shall do all in my power to help lose this superfluous envelope of fat that I've allowed to accumulate. I shall try to live as if I were slender and attractive. I ask the help of my subconscious to help me become my best self."

Add what you like about wanting to be popular or better looking or happier or more successful. But please make your demands all definite, and all good——and all personal for you. This isn't the time to be altruistic! You can help other people all of the rest of the day. Now, you must help yourself.

After you've spoken to your subconscious, forget the whole thing! You've planted the idea. Then live, all day, as if you really were the person you'd like to be.

As far as your diet is concerned, you'll have to diet even more than will be necessary once you weigh the amount you should weigh. But, if your attitude is right, not only will the diet be less distasteful—it will actually be more helpful. Psychosomatically, you'll be doing all you can for yourself.

When you've learned the exercises you must do, you can add them to your regime. I assure you they're not strenuous. I loathe exercises, but the few I find I must do have become a pleasant part of my daily routine. They are neither hard nor long. If they were, I'm sure I wouldn't do them! Of course you can exercise more strenuously if you like. That's up to you. But your thoughts and your diet must be constructive.

I'm not trying to turn you into a dear little optimist, full of nothing but beautiful thoughts—though, at that, that wouldn't be half bad, these days. I am trying to convince you that if you think positive thoughts about growing slender, you will grow slender—if your actions suit your thoughts.

You'll find it impossible to eat a huge cream dessert when you realize, with all parts of your mind, that it is not for you as you'd like to be—as you are, actually, in your subconscious mind.

The last thing before you go to sleep at night, after you're in bed and the lights are off, again "address the subconscious." Even thank your subconscious, if you've had a successful day! And give directions for the day ahead—and for the night! There are those who believe that the subconscious accomplishes its best work while we sleep—while the conscious mind is at rest—for the subconscious mind does not sleep, as our dreams prove. Even if you don't dream, or don't remember your dreams, the subconscious mind is busy. So it might as well be busy constructively for you. The Psychology Record Company, at 673 So. Coronado Street, Los Angeles 5, California, is so convinced that the subconscious can receive instruction during sleep that it has made a series of records aimed to teach the subconscious while you are asleep. One of these records, Number 13, I believe, is on Normal Weight.

Experiments have shown that people are helped, when learning a foreign language, by "hearing" records while they sleep.

You may not need a record to help your subconscious. You may not need anyone to tell you, while you sleep, that you are growing thinner and better looking, and getting to feel better, too. Your directions to your subconscious before you go to sleep may be enough. Sound foolish? Not nearly as foolish as you may believe, without giving it a trial. After all, what have you got to lose?

"I am getting more slender every day. I want you to help me become the slender, healthy good-looking person that I should be. I know that I am really a slender and attractive and popular and successful person. Help me and I shall try in every way, with my conscious mind, to do all I can to become my better self."

Those probably will not be your words at all. But I think you know what I mean. Instruct your subconscious. Thank your subconscious. And then do the things that will help your subconscious achieve its part of the bargain, and you may start in by thanking God, too, if you're not already doing that. It's an idea!

CHAPTER 17

Drink
yourself fat

ALL THESE PAGES, and not one word about drinking! I can just hear a lot of you: "This book is just like the others! Lots of words about eating—and nothing about drinking at all!" So, here, then, is a whole chapter about drinking. And I bet it isn't at all what the drinker wants to hear. Not if he wants to hear that he can drink all he wants and not gain a pound.

First of all, I want to say that I do not think that eating too much is like drinking too much. And I do not think that overweights need to form societies called "Eaters Anonymous" or "Fatties Anonymous[1]" or "Gluttons Anonymous" or anything else Anonymous. You who are too fat are going to think yourselves thin—and, I hope, have already started to think yourselves thin— without the assistance of any societies to help you, though you may join, with profit, such a society, if you are by nature a joiner, and are helped by group psychology.

If you want to belong to societies to stop this or start that, for gracious sakes don't let me stop you! If you want to belong to a society that will keep you from making pigs of yourselves, go ahead and join—with my

182

blessings. And I hope you have fun! All I mean is that I think you are smart enough, and have control enough of yourself, to get thin by yourself, with just the necessary help from your doctor and from whatever courses you find necessary—or just from your doctor and from this book, with whatever supplementary reading you find interesting and instructive. But excessive eating is not like excessive drinking at all. Ask your doctor!

If you drink too much, I'm all in favor of Alcoholics Anonymous. I think it's a grand organization and that it is doing swell work for those who need it. But as any alcoholic will tell you, alcoholism is a disease. An alcoholic is one who is allergic to alcohol. An alcoholic cannot drink at all. And there isn't anyone who can't eat at all. So you see the two conditions are not at all similar.

Alcoholics Anonymous have my great admiration and my hearty congratulations. But this chapter isn't for them at all! They aren't drinking—and I hope they will never drink. This is for the moderate drinker, who can take it or leave it alone. And I'm concerned only with getting you thin and fit. If you're an alcoholic, you've got to take care of yourself. That's too big a problem for me to tackle here.

First of all, I want to say that I don't drink. But then, I never did. I'm not allergic to alcohol. On New Year's Eve I'm likely as not to take a glass of champagne. I just don't like to drink! But if you do, there's no reason why you shouldn't if it doesn't hurt you. I go to cocktail parties; I serve drinks to my friends, if they

like to drink. Drinking is strictly up to you, although
the person who wants to diet is better off without alcohol. You've got to make up your own mind whether or
not you should drink—and when and how much.

All I can do about your drinking is to tell you what
effect alcohol will have on your diet—and give you the
caloric value of various drinks. They are high in carbohydrates. They contain no fat, very little protein or
vitamins—practically none, in fact, in most cases.

If you want to know more about alcohol and its effect on your diet than I can give you here, I recommend
The Fat Boy's Book, by Elmer Wheeler, published by
Prentice Hall, *How To Stop Killing Yourself,* by Dr.
Peter J. Steincrohn, published by Wilfred Funk, and that
fine textbook, *Nutrition and Diet in Health and Disease,*
by Dr. James S. McLester, published by W. B. Saunders,
which I've recommended to you before—and undoubtedly will recommend again and again.

Now let's get things straight about alcohol. It probably will not hurt you, if you're not an alcoholic—if
you're not allergic to alcohol. Alcohol is oxidized in the
body, and in small quantities may be used in metabolism to replace some carbohydrates or fat. In other
words, you may take some of it instead of your allowance of calories—but not of your protein calories. It
cannot, however, be depended on as the chief form of
nourishment because of this lack in its contents. Those
who are accustomed to it will oxidize a reasonable amount
in about seven hours. Those not accustomed to alcohol
will take twice that length of time.

Alcoholic drinks are taken for two reasons: for their flavor—and that seems odd to me, to whom they taste pretty terrible—or for the sense of well-being they produce. Doctors sometimes find alcoholic drinks are valuable in the treatment of certain diseases. For elderly persons and those with debilitating diseases they often have real value. They help, in these cases, in improving appetite and digestion. But folks who are too fat seldom have to have their appetites encouraged, nor do they need alcohol for digestion. Nervous indigestion, worry, anxiety and fatigue are known to be inhibiting, and alcohol removes the inhibiting influence and gives mental and physical relaxation. I hope that you don't need alcohol for any of these reasons.

Dr. Steincrohn estimates that there are 50,000,000 social drinkers in America, 3,000,000 excessive drinkers, and 750,000 who suffer from chronic alcoholism. He feels that moderate drinking is not harmful, and that an ounce or two of alcohol a day for elderly people may be beneficial. But he doesn't believe it is a cure-all for anything from a cold to a snake bite, though he frequently recommends one glass of sherry or one Martini before dinner, if you're tired or irritable.

So—one drink may be all right, even if you count the calories. Too many people, though, can't stop with that one drink. Look at your Beverage Table at the end of this chapter, and you'll see that a Martini averages about 130 calories. You'll have to decide for yourself if it is worth it to you to spend 130 of your daily calorie allowance on that one drink. And, of course, three Mar-

tinis mean 400 calories—or about half of the caloric
allowance of a strict diet—and not a bit of protein in that
400! A highball contains about 150 calories, if it's made
with either charged or plain water. And, of course,
alcohol mixed with a sweet beverage has even more
calories. Add about sixty calories more for a rum and coke,
or for one of those fattening drinks mixed with ginger
ale.

There's another difficulty, too, about drinking. If you're
on a diet that limits your liquid intake, you must count part
of those drinks as your liquid allowance. So, if you are on
a strict diet and want one Martini, you should drink it
quite a while before eating—an hour before dinner is best.
One cocktail an hour before dinner! Of course that doesn't
please you! Then cut out the cocktail.

Wine with dinner means more liquid—and more calories.
So look at your wine list before adding wine to your
dinner. Wine with dinner is an elegant and epicurean
custom. I'm sorry to say that you must limit it, if you
want to grow thin. One glass of very dry wine— at a
caloric count of 75 to 90 calories—may be added to your
dinner, if you insist on it. Go without your Martini and have
one glass of dry wine, if you enjoy it more.

A great many people on a diet solve the drinking
problem in another way. They allow themselves one
highball after dinner. They wait an hour after eating— and
then take, very leisurely, their one drink. Adding, of course,
that 150 calories. They enjoy that more than a midnight
snack.

The average man-about-town—or girl-about-town, if it comes to that—thinks nothing of, say, three cocktails before dinner, two glasses of wine with dinner, and at least three highballs after dinner. And that's little enough —if spaced over an evening at home or an evening at a night club. Sounds very festive? And very fattening. Fattening to the extent of about 1,000 calories—the exact amount of calories you're going to be allowed for your food expenditure for a whole day, unless your doctor gives you a different calorie limit.

It isn't only the drinks that fatten you, when you're at a cocktail party or a bar—or even at home. It's the things that go with them. Canapes, peanuts, crackers, tiny sandwiches and bits of sausage and bacon and olives can add up unbelievably. That caviar or salmon canape can easily amount to 50 or 75 calories. That bit of toast is 25 calories, and the piled-up cheese or caviar, red or black, or salmon or paté can have at least 25 calories more—and may add up to 50. Count 50 calories for one canape—and see what you get! A tiny sandwich is at least another 50 calories—25 or more for the tiny bite of bread, and 25 for the filling. Nuts count up quickly. A handful—and not too big a handful— count up to 100 calories. Olives, sweet pickles and other nibbles can easily add a hundred calories more. Three cocktails, a few canapes or nibbles—pretzels, cheese crackers, olives or nuts—and you've added seven or eight hundred calories—practically enough for a whole day's diet in that half hour before dinner!

What can you do?

"I can't cut my throat," you say. "I go to cocktail parties. I like them. I don't care too much about drinking, but I have to drink something."

I suppose you do. I don't. And I know a lot of other people who don't, too.

What can you drink?

You can order lemon and soda. And put a sweet tablet in it. Sucaryl, made by the Abbott Laboratories, is best, I think. It does not leave a bitter aftertaste. Tastes just like sugar, too. Each tablet has the value of one teaspoon of sugar. Two dropped into a glass of soda and lemon make a very good glass of lemonade. A poor substitute for a Martini? I'm sure! But it has very few calories and, outside of the liquid content, isn't bad for you. Or drink plain soda. It sounds revolutionary—but it isn't a bad idea. Tea or coffee, when you can get them—you can't always get them at cocktail parties—are all right, too. A small coke or a small ginger ale is about 65 calories—just about half of the caloric value of most alcoholic drinks. Not too satisfactory, if you're accustomed to something stronger—but you can get used to it. And feel so noble about it, too!

Plain cider, plain orange juice, plain grapefruit juice, plain pineapple juice or plain tomato juice are all good, if you can get them. Undoubtedly, though, you won't be satisfied with those mild substitutes. People might think you were on the wagon—and wouldn't that be terrible!

So, the best solution I can suggest is to order a small Sherry, a Dry Martini, or a Gibson on the Rocks, which is even dryer, they tell me, and make it last the whole period before dinner. While others drink and drink and drink, nibble and nibble and nibble, you can feel noble, with that one drink! And not be on the wagon. No one will question you. And you don't have to nibble, if you've got strength of character enough to stay away from the goodies.

At dinner, if you must, have your one glass of wine—very dry. But only if you've got to have it! Only if dinner would be dry and tasteless without it. If you can go without wine, so much the better. A lot of folks never have wine with dinner, you know—and live very well, too.

After dinner, you may be able to go without drinking at all. I don't know your habits. But, if you must drink, if you could limit your drinking to one highball, made with soda or plain water, you wouldn't be adding too many calories—and still you could feel that you were drinking.

You must cut out all " fancy" drinks—all drinks made with syrups or cream. They are far worse than your dry alcoholic beverages. I hate to think of the added calories that go into those eggnogs over the Christmas holidays—cream, eggs, half a dozen kinds of alcoholic drinks! Those "little lady" drinks, such as Alexanders, are on the *verboten* list, too. If you must drink, go in for the manly dry beverages!

Drinking may give you a feeling of well-being. And that's just fine. But drinking has another attribute. It gives you an appetite! You nibble peanuts, popcorn and canapes. And isn't that just what you need, when you're trying to limit your caloric intake! The dinner of herbs, I mean of salads, and vegetables and meat without added sauces, may taste fine if you're normally hungry, but after a couple of Martinis you'll crave richer viands—and reach for the Hollandaise sauce. Drinking takes off that top layer of inhibitions and makes you a bit reckless. To Hell with all those diet plans! What about an avocado pear, filled with rich dressing and crab meat as a first course, followed by a thick cream soup, steak, or maybe Veal Petronius—such good cheese sauce. And, of course, a couple of hot rolls, with a lot of butter, before the meal arrives, and maybe French fried potatoes with the meat, and a rich dessert, with a puff paste and whipped cream. My, I'm hungry just writing about it!

That's what happens, once you start to drink. Good resolutions fly out of the window. What to do? Well, start all over again the next morning. And learn to drink in moderation—and eat in moderation, too. Or maybe learn not to drink at all, if that's not asking too much. Maybe if you limit your drinking to that one Dry Martini before dinner, with the one highball afterward, you'll be able to manage. It's a good idea, anyhow.

Here, then, is your list. Maybe the sight of all of those calories will bring you to your senses. Here's hoping! Either way, here's to you! And to thinking yourself thin instead of drinking yourself fat.

BEVERAGE	Portion	Quantity	Alcohol	Total Extracts	Total Fuel Value	Calies per 100 Grams
			Per cent by Weight	Per cent.	Calories	Calories
A. DISTILLED LIQUORS.						
Brandy, California	Cordial.glass	20c.c	45.80	0.45	65	325
Brandy, cherry	"	20 "	44.00	.01	62	310
Brandy, cognac, pure French .	"	20 "	55.00	.02	78	300
Cocktail, Dry Martini	Cocktail glass	75 "	21.30	6.21	131	175
Gin	....	50 "	30.00	5.50	116	232

The enormous variation in the composition of alcoholic liquors has made it exceedingly difficult to choose values which should be accurate and comparable. As a rule, the percentages given are averages of a large number of analyses and if not strictly accurate are as nearly so as it is possible to obtain them.

When no authority is given, the figures are averages of those published by one or more authorities and cited by König.

The total extractives are reckoned as sugar, notwithstanding the fact that they comprise other substances than carbohydrates in small amounts which cannot be classed as foods. The percentage of these, however, is so small that the error is negligible.

Alcohol is computed solely on the basis of its function as a food. It must not be overlooked that in more than very moderate quantities it acts as a drug instead, and when taken to excess this action may negative entirely its action as a food, or even interfere with the digestion and absorption of other foods.

BEVERAGE	Portion	Quantity	Alcohol Per cent by Weight	Total Extracts Per cent.	Total Fuel Value Calories	Cal'ies per 100 Grams
A. DISTILLED LIQUORS—Continued						
liqueurs:						
Benedictine	Cordial glass	20 c.c.	42.40	35.00	88	440
Chartreuse.............	"	20 "	35.20	35.40	78	390
Curaçao	" "	20 "	42.00	27.90	82	410
Crème de Menthe.......	" "	20 –	36.50	28.28	74	370
Kümmel	" "	20 "	26.00	29.80	61	305
Rum.............	.....	50 "	43.50	.13	153	306
Rum, pure Jamaica	.....	50 "	69.61	.61	245	490
Whiskey, American, genuine .	.....	50 "	43.00	.70	152	304
Whiskey, European	.....	50 "	39.00	.....	137	274
B. WINES AND CIDERS.						
1. American Wines.						
California, red	Claret glass	120 "	9.50	3.10	95	79
California, white	" "	120 "	9.00	2.70	89	74
Sweet wines:						
Catawba	Sherry glass	30 –	11.07	5.60	30	100
Champagne.............	Champagne glass	30"	11.07	5.60	30	98
	Sherry glass	30 "	8.27	9.74	132	100
Port, California.......			14.81	12.17	53	176
Sherry, California.......	" "		11.67	5.53	38	126

BEVERAGE	Portion.	Quantity,	Alcohol. Per cent by Weight.	Total Extracts. Per cent.	Total Fuel Value. Calories	CaTies per 100 Grams.
B. WINES AND CIDERS—Continued.						
2. European Wines.						
Champagne, dry	Champagne glass	135 c.c.	10.42	2.36	112	83
French, red (claret)	Claret glass	120 "	8.16	2.42	81	67
French, white	" "	120 "	9.48	3.03	95	79
Mosel and Saar, white	" "	120 "	7.36	2.31	73	61
Rhein, white	" "	120 "	8.12	2.91	83	69
Sweet wines:						
Champagne	Champagne glass	135 "	9.50	12.88	161	119
Madeira	Sherry glass	30 "	15.40	5.52	39	130
Malaga	" "	30 "	11.93	21.73	52	173
Marsala	" "	30 "	15.85	5.28	40	133
Port	" "	30 –	16.69	8.05	45	150
Sherry	" "	30 w	17.45	3.98	42	140
Tokay, fresh	" "	30 w	11.19	12.72	39	130
3. Ciders.						
American, sweet	Glass	250 "	1.40	8.20	109	4
American, fermented		250 w	5.17	3.88		4

193

	Portion.	Quantity.	Alcohol.	Total Extracts	; Total Fuel Value	Cal'ies per 100 Grams.
			Per cent by Weight.	Per cent.	Calories	
C. MALT LIQUORS.						
1. American.						
Ale	Glass	250 c.c.	6.02	4.86	155	62
Lager beer, bottled........	"	250 "	4.53	4.96	130	52
Lager beer, draft...........	"	250 "	4.27	4.40	120	48
Porter........................	"	250 w	4.46	6.00	140	56
2. European.						
Ale	"	250 "	5.27	5.99	154	62
Bock Beer	"	250 w	4.20	7.10	146	58
Export beer.................	"	250 —	4.29	6.50	142	57
Light beer	"	250 w	3.69	5.39	120	48
Munich, heavy beer.........	"	250 "	4.54	9.96	182	73
Pilsen, export beer.........	"	250 *	4.28	4.69	123	49
Porter (Stout)	"	250 w	5.16	7.97	172	69
Weissbeer	"	250 n	2.79	5.29	103	41

The above table of alcoholic beverages is taken from Locke, Edwin A.: *Food Values*, and is published here through the courtesy of Appleton-Century-Crofts, Inc.

CHAPTER 18

The battle of
the bulge

EVERYBODY IS DIETING, THESE DAYS. Or practically everyone. That's the way it seems, anyhow. You can't go to a party without hearing of a couple of new diets or having someone produce a dog-eared slip of paper from purse or bill fold containing a diet a doctor has given him or her, or one that has been cut out of a paper or magazine.

Some of these diets are excellent. Some are old-fashioned or unscientific. All of them are supposed to produce wonderful results. Only a few are so badly balanced as to be actually harmful. There's one good thing about all of them. It doesn't matter much what they recommend. Why? I'll tell you—it's simple enough. Few diets are harmful, if followed for only a short period, for most of us have enough reserve energy in our systems to take care of us for a period of from three to eight weeks. We'll stay perfectly healthy for that length of time, living on our own body, providing there is no infection or serious toxic protein loss. On a badly balanced diet, we'd be out of luck after that length of time. But

195

few people pursue those trick diets longer than a few weeks.

You'll get your own special diet in the very next chapter. But I hope you realize, by now, that diet alone, without proper preparation—without the proper mental attitude—is not going to do what it's supposed to do, and is not going to help you over a long period of time. Your diet, with the proper changes, which you'll learn about, too, will help you for as long as you stay on it— and I hope you will stay on it. That is, if, by the time you start it, you are ready for it. You certainly should be! But don't, I beg of you, copy it off and hand it around, or try to put your friends on it. Apart from the other things you must do—the exercises which you'll learn about, the things I hope you've already learned—it won't work. Not as a magic get-thin-quick diet, anyhow! It's just an integral part of the way you think yourself thin.

Carl Malmberg, in his excellent book, *Diet and Die,* published by Hill-Curl, has written an expose of some of the more ridiculous diets. Many "recommended" diets show a lack of knowledge of psychology, digestion, metabolism, nutrition and the functions of the human body. Not that all published diets are bad. On the contrary— some are good, and good for you, and are accompanied by excellent and helpful advice. But if you don't know about foods and about the human body, you're apt to go wrong.

Many movie stars of a previous generation suffered serious upsets as a result of those bad diets. A few died

Others became dangerously ill. Now, Hollywood has, for the most part, learned not to go on diets without medical supervision.

One actress became very ill on a diet of lemon juice and raw vegetables and raw fruit. Another added black coffee to that same diet—and was just as ill.

Others, wanting to get thin in a hurry, added bran to their reduced diets, "for roughage." They got roughage —and a bad case of stomach trouble at the same time. Intestinal irritation, indigestion and colitis can result from too much roughage. So don't add bran or any other roughage to your diet without medical supervision.

If I say one word against a vegetarian diet, I'll get letters from dozens of vegetarians saying I don't know what I'm talking about. I can't even tell you not to go on a vegetable diet without your doctor's advice, because most vegetarians don't believe in doctors, either, so that recommendation will be just as displeasing to them. However, I find that most vegetarians are not vegetarians in the true sense—they add fruit, eggs, milk, butter and cheese to their diet, making it a good, well-balanced diet, but not at all a vegetarian diet, in a narrow sense. Vegetables are wonderful food, but to my way of thinking they must be supplemented by such foods as milk, eggs, cheese, high-protein cereals, and even meat and fish.

Some animals live wholly on vegetable foods—the horse, the cow, the sheep and the goat, for example. These herbivorous animals have long, capacious intestines, with a large pouch, the caecum, where grass and hay can be digested. Carnivorous—meat-eating—animals have a much shorter digestive tract, and are unable to digest grasses at all. Man's digestive tract lies in between these two types—his intestines are of moderate length, and he can digest a non-bulky mixed diet, which, it seems to most scientists, he ought to have. Read Dr. L. Jean Bogert's *Diet and Personality,* with its subtitle, "Fitting Food to Type and Environment," published by Macmillan—especially the chapter on the food faddist, if you're interested in pursuing this subject. Personally, I believe in a high-protein diet, both for reduction and for health, which is not always possible on a true vegetarian diet.

Professor Chittenden at Yale University believed in a low-protein diet, and conducted some interesting but not-at-all-conclusive experiments—and ever since then, everyone who believes in a low-protein diet has been quoting him—without knowing what he was attempting to prove. All he did prove, it seems *to* me, was that one can live on a low-protein diet for a short time. Practically all of the men in Chittenden's experiment returned to their former eating habits, once the short experiments were over. I still believe in a high-protein diet, which all of the later scientists seem to agree is far better.

Gayelord Hauser's books are among the best for laymen, and preach some excellent health habits. But I don't approve of his vegetable salt and potassium broth —because they are expensive for what you get, and contain more salt than I consider good for a reducing diet. And I don't believe in as much laxative as his Swiss Kriss gives you. I also think he overestimates the good qualities of molasses. But on the whole, I think you'll get a lot of good out of Hauser's books—his new *Look Younger, Live Longer,* as well as *The Gaylord Hauser Cook Book,* which I'll refer to again. You'll do better following the Hauser theories than you will following most of the diets recommended by less informed writers. They're interesting and well balanced, for the most part —and contain meat as well as eggs and fruit and vegetables.

One of the worst diets ever foisted on the public is the Hollywood Eighteen Day Diet. This was once so popular that you could get it in any restaurant, by just mentioning what day of the diet you were on. Supposedly sponsored first by a California citrus fruit company, and now by a cracker company, it is still around. Like most other diets, it won't hurt you for eighteen days. It is, however, deficient in proper nutritive elements. One day's breakfast consists of one-half of a grapefruit, one slice of Melba toast and coffee without cream or sugar. For luncheon, you get the other half of the grapefruit, one egg, a bit of raw vegetable and again toast and coffee, and for dinner, meat, salad, grapefruit and coffee. You'll lose on it, of course. But you can do better!

The pineapple and lamb chop diet was started by a reputable physician in order to give a Hollywood star a diet she would enjoy.

"Choose any meat and any fruit you like," he told her. She chose pineapple and lamb chops.

"That's your diet!" he said. Curiously enough, it's a good diet—high in protein, low in carbohydrates. You'll reduce on it. The only thing the matter with it is that it is monotonous. You can chose any one meat, and any one vegetable or fruit, and make up your own diet— and you'll probably do just as well with it. For a long haul, I don't think you'll like it too well.

In spite of the pretty advertising that ran some time ago grape juice is not reducing. All food is fattening, you know—and there's nothing in grape juice that even helps reduction in any way. It contains sugar—and sugar is fattening. It is pleasant to drink, not at all harmful, and can be substituted for any other fruit drink. If you count the calories, and take grape juice as part of your fruit calories, you'll do very well with it. To think that, *per se,* it will reduce you, is just part of the Fool's Paradise of advertising.

The baked potato and skimmed milk diet is another flimsy diet that you can omit with pleasure. A baked potato is fine, occasionally. It contains minerals and some proteins, along with starch, and, if eaten with enough meat, is good for you. Skimmed milk is a fine, well balanced food—and is included in most diets. But together they do not form a balanced diet. For a few days, if you want to feel like a martyr, it won't hurt you—and you'll certainly lose weight on it.

Tomatoes and hard boiled eggs constitute another two-piece diet that has its enthusiastic followers. It is fairly well balanced, and high in proteins and the nutrients you need, and you're supposed to lose your appetite on it—another way to get thin—but like all diets of this sort, it is monotonous.

Grapefruit and steak is one of the better tasting of these two-piece affairs. With steak at the price it is today, the grapefruit and steak adherents have the advantage of feeling luxurious while they are half starved. Try it if you like. Like the other two-piece meals, it won't hurt you. Not as long as you'll stay on it, I'm sure.

The bread and butter diet is one of the least satisfactory of these limited regimes. However, if you get starved for fresh bread—and often, on a diet, bread-hunger does develop, you may enjoy this bread and butter eating for a few days. The bread can be fresh or toasted, the butter sweet or salted. Nothing else! Just bread and butter! You break the charm and spoil the results if you add to it.

The banana and skimmed milk diet is still popular. Curiously enough, it was actually invented by Dr. George A. Harrop, of Johns Hopkins University, and was published in the Journal of the American Medical Association, and then taken up by the United Fruit Company. This diet has two parts, each running from ten days to two weeks. The first part consists of four to six ripe bananas, and from three to four glasses of skimmed milk, with enough vegetables to prevent constipation, each day. The second half adds lean meat, eggs and fish. You're likely to lose on the first half, but not much on the second, and you can then repeat the process under your doctor's supervision.

You can find various forms of liquid diets in nearly every diet book—and they are recommended by dozens of people. These usually consist of fruit juices and milk, drunk alternately. These liquid diets are given various names by their sponsors. They aren't at all bad—and a liquid diet, one day each week, is recommended by many doctors. Grapefruit juice, pineapple juice, orange juice, tomato juice and milk are usually the recommended liquids. You choose your own, and drink about eight glasses of the liquids during the day, at any intervals you find convenient. If your doctor recommends them, you might try liquid diets occasionally.

Diet and Health With Key to the Calories, by Dr. Lulu Hunt Peters, with revisions by Eloise Davison, Director of the New York Herald Tribune Home Institute, is a good book on reduction and contains some helpful and amusing reading matter. My chief objection to this book is that the calories are chosen without much reference to whether they are protein, fat or carbohydrate. But you'll lose—and you'll lose sensibly enough on these diets—and I think you'll find the book interesting.

Sensible Dieting, by Dr. William Engel, with the Engel vital calorie diets, published by Alfred Knopf, is one of the better diet books. The diets are well balanced and arranged in detail according to the seasons, and the chapters devoted to a discussion of foods are well and sensibly written. I think you'll enjoy this especially if you want more diet lists.

You Can Live Longer Than You Think¡ by Daniel C. Munro, is a fine book, with chapters on reduction that you'll like, I'm sure. Dr. Munro believes in a high-protein diet and gives some good high-protein menus. His book is one of the best. An interesting chapter lists the longevity of the Biblical characters—all of whom, according to Dr. Munro, lived on meat diets.

Your Weight and How to Control It, published by Doubleday, and edited by Dr. Morris Fishbein, Editor of *The Modern Home Medical Adviser* and *The Popular Medical Encyclopedia,* contains over a dozen chapters on various aspects of overweight, each chapter by an expert. I think you'll be especially interested in "Good Habits and Weight," by Martha F. Trulson, Ethel D. Walsh and Dr. Frederick J. Stare, "Fads in Weight Reduction," by Dr. Fishbein, and "Success in Reducing," by Ann Delafield.

One of the first books on diet was *Eat and Grow Thin¡* with a preface by Vance Thompson, and with excellent menus. Published in 1914 by Dutton, this is out of print, but it isn't too hard to find second-hand copies. Curiously enough, although there isn't any mention of the newer reduction methods, it is as up-to-date as if it had been published today. The menus are well selected, the recipes excellent. The dinners are a bit over-crowded—for they were written in a day when we thought we had to have more things to eat. One dinner included mussels mariniere, dolmas, broiled mushrooms, roast fowl with aspic jelly, coleslaw and stewed apples. Another dinner is oysters, fish, roast guinea-fowl with pickled walnuts, mashed turnips, pineapple salad and gelatin. You get the idea! But all of the items mentioned are low in calories and high enough in proteins, so, with proper eliminations, the menus can be used satisfactorily, and the preface is sensible and well written. *You Can Be Thin,* a method to achieve slenderness through psychology, by Dr. Herman Friedel, with a foreword by Dr. Milton Jacovy, published by Caxton House, is a sensible book on reduction, and contains the University of Illinois reduction menus, of 1,000 calories per day. Here are one day's menus:

BREAKFAST:

25 grapes; coddled egg; 2 slices bacon; whole milk; coffee.

DINNER:

Roast chicken, 3 thin slices; cranberry sauce, 1 tablespoon; cauliflower, 1/4 small head; string beans, 1/2 cup; head of lettuce, 1 large serving, with 3/4 tablespoon French dressing.

SUPPER:

Cold sliced chicken, 2 small slices; celery and carrot sandwich, small; 1 sliced orange; 1 glass of whole milk.

Do you like ice cream? A lot of people do. And they hate to go without it, just because they are trying to reduce. Marion White, the author of *Sweets Without Sugar,* has taken care of that for you—she shows how to get thin, and eat ice cream. It doesn't seem possible, but Miss White proves it. Her book, *Ice Cream Diets,* published by M. S. Mill, gives you ice cream twice a day. She also gives some good recipes, which I'll tell you about, later on. Here are one day's menus, as given by Miss White:

BREAKFAST:
Orange juice, 1 cup (90 calories); 1 slice buttered toast (75 calories); tea or coffee.

LUNCHEON:
Egg and lettuce sandwich, no butter (170 calories); ice cream, 2/3 cup (200 calories).

DINNER:
Vegetable soup, 1 1/2 cups (80 calories); 1 lamb chop, fat removed (150 calories); 1 baked potato (100 calories); 1 pat butter (100 calories); 1/2 cup peas (65 calories) ; ice cream, 2/3 cup (200 calories) ;Total for the day 1,130 calories.

Victor Lindlahr's popular book, *Eat and Reduce,* is now reprinted by Permabooks at 35 cents—and should be in every reducer's library. It gives lists of foods, with food values and very good menus. Here are the menus for a day:

BREAKFAST:
Orange; a second fruit; coffee; 1/2 cup milk. (This is standard, the same every day.)

LUNCHEON:
Tomato and lettuce salad; mashed turnips; string beans; peaches.

DINNER:

Watercress and onion salad; mutton chop; asparagus; pineapple.

The weight and caloric value of each food is given each day. Here is a sensible book, with few fads, with which you can reduce painlessly.

One of the most popular books ever published on reduction—it must be in its twentieth printing by now—is *Eat and Get Slim* by Donald G. Cooley, published by Wilfred Funk. There are chapters on calories, on vitamins, and on good looks and charm. The daily menus, showing how much you're supposed to lose each month, give a 1,000-calorie diet, complete with the carbohydrate, protein, fat and total calorie content of each article on the menus. The book is well arranged and comprehensive. Here are one day's menus:

BREAKFAST:

1/2 grapefruit; cold ham, no fat; 1 shirred egg; large graham cracker; black coffee or clear tea.

LUNCHEON :

1 cup consommé; serving of beef or calves' liver, pan broiled; bacon, broiled crisp, 2 slices; spinach, 1/2 cup; tomato and lettuce salad; 1 glass skim milk; black coffee or clear tea.

DINNER :

1 cup beef broth; pot roast, average serving; salad, egg and tomato; 1 orange; black coffee or clear tea.

The Low-Fat, Low-Cholesterol Diet, What to Eat and

How to Prepare It, by E. Virginia Dobbin, Dr. Helen F. Gofman, Helen C. Jones, Lenore Lyon and Clare-Beth Young, with introductions by Drs. Thomas P. Lyon and John W. Gofman, published by Doubleday, is a valuable diet book for those who are interested in reducing the cholesterol content of their food. It has been proved that cholesterol is found in highly concentrated form in parts of the arteries which are afflicted with arteriosclerosis. A great many doctors believe that an upset in the body's capacity to handle cholesterol and fats properly will result in hardening of the arteries. Other doctors believe that cholesterol is formed, whether or not it is included in the diet. Your own doctor will have to decide for you. Either way, the new book is excellent because the recipes are practically fat-free—and a great many of them are low in caloric values. All of the calorie values are given. So if you hunt for the right recipes, you'll get a great deal out of the book. The recipes are interesting, and those I tested have a good flavor.

Dr. Alfred L. George has written a good book, *Your Weight and Your Life,* published by Norton.

There are a lot of other books on diet, but I think you'll find these the most satisfactory, as far as your needs are concerned. People who want to reduce are seldom satisfied with one person's advice. And why should they be? Getting thin is a serious business. The person with a small bookshelf—not necessarily a Five-Foot Bookshelf—of reduction literature can get an over-all view of obesity, and have a good time comparing the advice, and experimenting with the menus.

The magazines are as prolific as the book publishers in giving diet advice. Perhaps the best known is the *Harper's Bazaar* Diet, which has been reprinted by *Harper's Bazaar,* and by the *Hearst Publications.* It is complete, with excellent advice and menus. Here are one day's menus:

BREAKFAST :
   1/2 grapefruit; cup of black coffee.
LUNCHEON :
   Minute steak; stewed tomatoes.
DINNER :
   Steak; stewed tomatoes; lettuce and tomato salad; plain spinach.

You may get tired of these diets—and they wouldn't do, for a protracted period—but for ten days, which is how long the routine is supposed to continue, you'll lose weight satisfactorily.

In *Good Housekeeping,* Maxine Davis wrote one of her excellent articles on obesity, treating it from the psychological angle, and giving fine advice.

One of the best articles ever published was Elizabeth Woody's "Eat Well and Lose Weight," in *Holiday,* later reprinted by that magazine. This was based on Dr. George H. Gehrmann's experiments as Medical Director at E. I. duPont de Nemours and Company. You can get a copy of this by sending ten cents to *Holiday,* in Philadelphia. The diet is high-protein, and consists of three meals, each with fat meat and one low-carbohydrate accompaniment—even potatoes, if you want them. A fine diet, and one that should receive serious consideration.

Hygeia, the Health Magazine of the American Medical Association, has published a number of fine articles on weight reduction. Some of these have been reprinted, and you may like to have them. Four of them are: *How to Reduce,* by Maurice Hardgrove; *Let the Scales Check Your Calories,* by Amalia Lauta; *Can You Take It or Leave It,* by Phoebe M. Walters; and *100-Calorie Portions of Common Foodstuffs,* by the Bureau of Health Education.

Clementine Paddleford, the excellent food expert, will keep you up to date on new foods and new menus for reducers. Practically every week she finds valuable additions to the dieter's menu. Dorothy Kilgallen, Leonard Lyons, Danton Walker—most of the syndicated columnists—are constantly publishing new ideas for dieters. A lot of them are worth trying.

Josephine Lowman in the *New York Post,* Alma Archer in the *Daily Mirror,* and Antoinette Donnelly in *The News* have all written excellent series of articles on weight reduction, together with advice and menus. And in dozens of other newspapers throughout the country, feature writers have written well and understandingly on the subject. Even the *New York Times, m* its Magazine Section, has devoted articles to reduction and to low-calorie recipes.

Walter Winchell has never given advice on diet, but

he has helped many people by praising them after they lost weight and improved their appearance.

Mary Margaret McBride includes, among her radio sponsors, an excellent high-protein, low-calorie bread, salmon and other reduction helps.

There are, too, throughout the country, the various health farms for reduction. Those for men go in for strenuous exercise and large steaks. Those for the women, as nearly as I can find out, serve liquid diets and give massage and some exercise. You get milk and fruit juice, and to me they sound deadly dull. I may be wrong. Certainly they are most profitable—for the people who run them. I don't see why anyone should take out the time to go away from home to be on a liquid diet. Surely, any woman can develop enough strength of character to stick to such a diet at home, if she felt it necessary, though there are other diets that serve just as well, and which might be a bit more palatable and less monotonous.

With all of this help, there's no need to weigh too much. You may not need all of them. Nor even any of them. Your own special diet is just ahead. With it and with any other of these you want as an occasional diet, for variety—you'll be well taken care of.

Dr. H. L. Marriott of Great Britain, in the *British Medical Journal,* describes a diet in which you can eat as much as you like. Considering British food problems, perhaps this isn't as generous as it seems. Dr. Marriott doesn't believe in counting calories but in eating and drinking as much as you like, or can get, of lean meats, poultry, game, live fish (not canned), eggs, potatoes, all other vegetables cooked without fat, fruits of all kinds, not dried or canned, sour pickles, clear soups, salads without oil, salt, pepper, mustard and vinegar. No fats, oils, cream, sugar, jam, sweets, puddings, ices, nuts, cake, pastries, cereals, cheese or alcohol are allowed. This diet was published in *Your Life Magazine,* and drew a lot of attention. It seemed too generous to be true. When you study it, you find it doesn't differ a great deal from other diets—it just seems to be different.

My idea for a diet is a bit more definite. Not an iron-clad rule of exactly what you must eat and when—but a prescribed outline, so you'll know how much food you should have, and the best quality of the foods you need. It won't be such a terrible diet, I promise you!

CHAPTER 19

Try this for size

HERE, THEN, IS YOUR DIET. Tailored especially for you. It is not a miracle diet, for the reason that I'm no magician. And neither is anyone else I've been able to locate. So if you're going around looking for magic, I'm afraid you're out of luck in this second half of the Twentieth Century.

This diet will reduce you. It will reduce you easily and pleasantly and without pain. You'll be well fed— undoubtedly better fed than you've been for some time —for the fact that you're overweight means that you've been over and not well fed, that you have been eating the wrong things—for you.

I could give you a diet that would reduce you far more quickly. In other words, it would be a starvation diet. You'd be eating up your own fat at a greater rate —and not getting the nutrition that you ought to have.

But this diet doesn't stand alone! It isn't the sort of diet you'll want to tear out or copy and carry in your pocket and give to your friends in exchange for their diet.

This diet depends on *you* for its success *for* you. Of course you'd get thin if you just followed it and did

nothing more. You'll get thin quicker and more comfortably—and more permanently—if, by now, you understand the reasons you're fat and are trying to overcome your wrong living habits, and wrong thoughts—if
you are working with your subconscious.

This diet is part of your life. It is a permanent diet.
Of course, after you've reached your perfect weight,
you can add to it to keep that weight. This diet is part
of your way of life. It must be accompanied by the right
thoughts, the right actions. In other words, you're
really to think yourself thin—and stay thin because of
your own thoughts. Thinking, proper exercise, proper
diet, proper living—these will make you a well-rounded, fine person, who looks and feels well, and who is
able to get the most out of life—and live for a longer
time, too.

Your medical examination: Have you had that yet?
You're not to start on this diet—on any diet, if you
take my advice—until you've had the medical examination I advised in Chapter 10. If your doctor approves
of this diet—and he probably will—you're to follow it.
If he doesn't—because of some allergy or some physical variance in you—you're to follow his advice. He
may change this diet a little to suit you better.

Your medication: You're not to take any medicine
at all without your doctor's thorough examination and
prescription. You may need glandular medication—
though I doubt it. Your doctor will prescribe it for you,
if you do. You probably will need a vitamin and mineral supplement with your diet, though this diet is un-

THINK YOURSELF THIN

usually rich in vitamins and minerals. But today's foods are, unfortunately, sometimes denatured. You don't get your vegetables and fruits as soon as they're plucked at the farm—and some of the nutrition is lost. Ask your doctor about this.

The vitamin supplements routinely added to certain diets are pharmaceutical preparations—tablets or capsules of a composition approximately that of the "hexa-vitamin tablet" of the Pharmacopaeia of the United States. They contain:

Thiamine hydrochloride (vitamin Bi)—2 mg.

Riboflavin (vitamin B2)—3 mg.

Ascorbic acid (vitamin C)—75 mg.

Vitamin A—5,000 LU.

Vitamin D—400 LU.

Added yeast, preferably in the form of flocculent dried brewers' yeast, is especially desirable where a full complement of the B-complex vitamins is desired. The usual dose is one ounce—2 rounded tablespoonfuls—mixed with liquid, such as water, milk, soup, tomato juice or fruit juice. Personally, I prefer yeast tablets. You can swallow them right down, without any bother at all. Even my little dog likes them, and Dr. James R. Kinney, Chief Veterinarian at the Ellen Prince Speyer Hospital, says that they're good for dogs, too—especially city dogs, whose diets sometimes lack proper vitamins.

Ask your doctor about the use of mineral oil. Today, doctors are finding that it doesn't destroy any real amount of vitamins, and is non-habit-forming. If your doctor approves of it, you can use it in salad dressings —see my special recipes—and for frying—a luxury usually denied people on diets, because of the fat used.

Some doctors also prescribe Milk of Magnesia as a laxative while you're dieting. I don't think you'll need it, if you eat properly. But I like and use mineral oil— and find it a great help in adding oils to dressings and cooking, especially when it is mixed with small quantities of olive and cooking oils.

Salt and water: Your diet will probably be more effective if you limit your salt and water intake. In fact, a lot of people lose weight by this method alone—a sort of dehydration. I don't approve of losing too much weight in this way—and none at all unless you have your doctor's approval. This consists of taking *no* water with your meals—and very little liquids. Dry meals! You'll get used to them. Don't drink for about an hour before you eat—and for about an hour afterwards. Your food will digest better. It will taste just as good, once you get used to it. I used to be the hostess' annoyance by drinking glass after glass of water at meals. I was fat, too! Now I never drink at meals—and even go slow on soups or too-wet accompaniments—and I feel just fine. Look better, too! Four glasses of water—of liquid—a day could be enough for you.

Salt should not be omitted altogether. Your system needs salt. And in hot weather you'll need even more salt than usual. But, on the whole, you can cut down your salt allowance, for salt is not fattening per se, but it holds water. Read Chapter 6 again, for more about salt.

Alcohol: You learned about alcohol and diet in Chapter 17. This is just a sort of review—summing up. And you know, now, how fattening alcohol can be.

You'll be better off if you stop drinking altogether. You'll lose weight more easily—feel better, too. Unless you're old and your doctor insists that you need alcohol —and that isn't likely, either—my advice is to give up all alcohol for the most successful think-yourself-thin regime.

"Oh, so that's it! You're one of those kill-joys!" I can hear you say. "I thought you were different. That I could drink and still follow your advice." So you can —if you insist on it. I bow to custom, to your own peculiar tastes. If you insist—I repeat—*if you insist*—you may have two drinks a day! I don't advise it. I don't encourage it. But, if you feel that it adds to your well-being, if it makes you more comfortable and happier, then have your two drinks. More than that, and you're not on a think-yourself-thin program—you're on your own—and I promise nothing.

Your first drink may be a very dry Martini or other dry drink, taken at least one hour before dinner! If you take it nearer to your dinner than that, it will give you too much liquid in your stomach for your diet to be most effective and, what is much worse, it will stimulate your appetite—make you reckless and want to eat more and forget all about your plans for looking and feeling better and losing weight. You're better off without that first drink, unless you actually need it as a pick-me-up. Some older people actually need some alcohol for quick energy. But why not get accustomed to going without alcohol—the "glass crutch" that isn't going to do you a great deal of good? I won't say another word! I won't have the liquor industry banging on my door!

Your second drink—or your first drink, if you've done without that cocktail—could be one glass of very dry wine with your dinner—if you are happier with wine at dinner and are accustomed to it. Again, you're better off without it. It gives liquid in your stomach that you don't need, and it stimulates your appetite. It's wonderful for that—and folks on diets do not need appetite-stimulators. *Au contraire,* as we never say.

If you haven't had your two drinks, and still insist on your quota of alcohol, you may have one highball, or its equivalent, after dinner, one hour after eating. This is the least harmful drink of the day—if you can limit it to one drink. It may add to the pleasure of your evening. I get a lot of pleasure out of my evenings without it. It also adds 150 calories to your diet. Use your own judgment, your own strength of will. You must count every drink as part of your food allowance. Some old people think they need this drink.

There are, of course, to be no nibbles of extras with any of your drinks. No salted nuts! No pretzels! No canapes! No potato chips! Count every bite as part of your food allowance.

Appetite Depressors: Your doctor will undoubtedly give you some. Sometimes they work. Sometimes they prove useless. There are a lot of patent ones on the market, too. Not to be taken without your doctor's prescription! You may prefer a piece of candy. One piece! Preferably a small piece of hard candy, slowly dissolved in the mouth. Some people say it helps them lose their appetite—the sugar makes them feel satisfied with less food. "Takes the edge off." Other people find that a piece of candy eaten right after a low-calorie meal gives them a feeling of fullness, of satisfaction, that nothing else can give them. You should be able to go without sweets—but few people on diets ever do.

Funny, sugar is the one thing that all specialists frown on. Dentists say it is bad for the teeth. Specialists on diets say it makes fat and has only one virtue—just high carbohydrates, which give quick energy. And yet the candy shops flourish, and bring out luscious new goodies every year. I asked a candy manufacturer why he didn't make a candy that was low in calories and full of some of the less-fattening fruits—maybe sugar substitutes and gelatin and dry skimmed milk—such as dieters are always experimenting with at home. I believe he turned pale, under his expensive Palm Beach tan.

"Don't say such a thing!" he groaned. "Don't you see what you'd be doing? You'd be reminding everyone who saw non-fattening candy that other candy was fattening. It might ruin the candy industry." He shuddered and turned away. So you'll never buy any non-fattening candy at your favorite candy shops—just high-calorie goodies which are on your "don't touch" list. Too bad! Of course, you can get very decent substitutes at the health-food shops. More about those later. Or you can make your own sweets. More about that, too. Candy is one of the sacrifices you'll have to make for health and appearance. Count your candy calories as part of your food allowance.

Benzedrine and Dexedrine are the best known appetite depressors. Taken half an hour before meals, they work splendidly with some people—and not at all with others. Certainly they should not be taken without your doctor's consent. In Hollywood, a lot of busy people live on a diet composed largely of Benzedrine, it seems to me. Not for reduction, but for energy! It frequently does give energy, and frequently more serious trouble. Be careful of Benzedrine! Newer appetite depressors are being prescribed by physicians, too. Some of them actually do depress appetites. I've tried a lot of them. They do not depress my appetite. I can eat just as heartily after I take one of them as before. I like to eat! I have to do all my own appetite curbing, without benefit of drugs. Easy to do? I'm not sure. I am sure it's worth doing.

R.D.X., made by the Lo-Calory Food Corporation, is an appetite depressor made of skimmed milk powder, dextrose, ascorbic acid and a couple of other ingredients. R.D.X. tablets have a fairly pleasant lemony taste. They won't hurt you—and they are low in calories. A friend of mine swears by them. They may help you.

Ayds, made by the Campana Corporation, are a "mineral and vitamin candy," used as an appetite depressor, and must, of course, be taken along with a non-fattening diet. These contain, among other things, corn syrup, sweetened whole milk, vegetable oil, soya flour, powdered egg yolk and vitamins. They taste like—and are —a sort of caramel. They may serve you well as an appetite depressor—a low-calorie, vitamin-fortified sweet. They certainly cannot harm you in any way, and if you find a sweet helps you, they are better than unfortified candy. They contain about thirty calories a caramel, I believe. The average caramel has about 50 calories— and of course does not have as much vitamin or mineral content. You must remember to count the calories.

One of the best commercial products is Protam, a "nutritional supplement for a low-calorie reducing regiment This, too, must be taken along with a careful diet. Protam is manufactured by the Protam Corporation, and has a 44% protein content and contains 26% carbohydrates. It does contain cotton-seed flour, protein hydrolysate and valuable vitamins. It is a powder, to be taken in hot liquids, and may help you.

The skimmed milk tablets manufactured by the American Dietaids Company are not made especially as an appetite depressor, but they are an excellent between-meal tidbit. They contain all of the excellent nutriments of skimmed milk, are only about seven calories in food value, and are as good as anything I can think of, if you feel you must be nibbling on something and don't want to yield to a high-calorie sweet.

All diet depressors are crutches—but you may need one of them when you're starting on your diet. They may actually be good for you—mentally as well as physically, You may not need them at all. Talk it over with your doctor. And use your own good judgment.

Exercise: You'll exercise for ten minutes night and morning, as part of your think-yourself-thin regime. It won't be too bad! You may enjoy it. You might even go in for more strenuous exercise, if you can take it. More about exercise in Chapter 23. In fact, it's all about exercise.

If someone gave me a certain amount of money each day—and I wish someone would—and I knew I shouldn't spend more than that much, but could get along well with it if I were careful, I'd be a fool if I didn't spend it wisely. Unfortunately, no one is giving me any money to spend— nor can I pass any along to you, so the simile isn't too apt. So you must stretch your imagination a bit and pretend that you're being given a thousand calories to spend each day. The catch is, you'll have to pay for them yourself, more than likely! Anyhow, you have the thousand calories for food every day. Shouldn't you make the best of them—spend them as wisely as possible?

On 1,000 calories, or even a few more, you can reduce very nicely—no matter how those calories are used. You can waste them on food! that won't help you. Or you can distribute them wisely throughout the day—on foods that will make you look well, and keep you well.

While you're dieting, you must tell yourself that you can have everything to eat you want, as long as you keep within that calorie range—or go just a little outside of it. If you wanted to spend the whole amount on cocktails, you'd still reduce—but wouldn't you be a fool to do it? If, after you dieted a while, you got very hungry for baked beans or chocolate creams or lemon pie, you could diet most of the day and then spend your 1,000 calories on your peculiar delicacy. I knew a movie star who loved chocolate creams. Once a week she didn't eat a thing until around ten o'clock at night. Then she retired for the night—with ten luscious chocolate creams —and very slowly munched them all. I know of another actress who munches chocolates—and spits them out. Not a very dainty thing to do for such a dainty girl. She realizes that she necessarily swallows some of them, so about once a week she goes on a "secret vice orgy" with her box of chocolates. Ridiculous? Maybe so. But the girls diet carefully all of the rest of the week. Much better, of course, if they trained their appetites so that they enjoyed the right foods all the time.

For you can train your appetite. That is certain. You can train yourself to enjoy foods with their natural flavors and only a little salt or salt substitute. You can train yourself away from chocolates, away from alcohol. You can train yourself away from fat foods, poultry stuffing, corn bread, hot biscuits, jams, jellies, preserves, syrups, cakes, candy, cookies, pastries, salted nuts, all "nibbles" at cocktail time, high-caloried hominy, macaroni, noodles and spaghetti, gravies, rich sauces, baked beans—except soy beans—pies, the richer cheeses, too much bread, too many crackers, fattening fruits —yes, there are such things—all high-caloried, concentrated foods. What is left for you? As if you didn't know! All lean meats—even ham, when it isn't too fat, chopped meats, steaks, stews, roasts, and especially kidneys, sweetbreads, liver, brains, tripe, chicken, practically all fish except the fattest varieties, shrimps, oysters, lobster, crab meat, and all of the low-caloried vegetables and fruits given in Chapter 12. Other things too—skimmed milk, buttermilk, yogurt, when made with skimmed milk, cottage cheese, pot cheese, farmer's cheese, the cheese mixtures given in my recipes, high gluten breads, crackers and spaghetti and macaroni, and the health foods you'll learn about. Plenty to eat—if you use your brains. Yes, you'll have to think yourself thin.

For your 1,000 calories, this is what you should eat: 70 to 75 grams of protein; about 40 grams of fat; about 100 grams of carbohydrates. You also should have about 850 mg. of Calcium and n or 12 mg. of Iron, as well as the vitamins needed for your system—around 7,000 I.U. of Vitamin A; 1.4 mg. of Thiamine; 1.7 mg. of Riboflavin; 11 mg. of Niacin and 180 mg. of Ascorbic Add. The vitamins and minerals are needed to keep you well and young—and can be supplemented; the carbohydrates are mainly for satiety—so that you'll feel you have enough to eat. Fats are restricted because you'll probably gain weight if, on a mixed diet, you eat too many of them. The proteins should be of good quality—in the form of eggs, meat, milk and cheese, helped along with even more proteins from vegetables, fruit and cereals and gelatin—which become more valuable when they are mixed with the good grade of protein.

What does this all mean? It means that you may have coffee and tea—which are without caloric value—if you sweeten them with one of the non-caloric sweeteners; about two thin slices of whole wheat, gluten or enriched bread a day; about one or two teaspoonfuls of butter; skimmed milk; desserts from your milk, fruit and egg allowance; about 30 grams of carbohydrates in fruit; 150 grams or more of meat, eggs and cheese; 12 grams of carbohydrates in fresh vegetables; soups, when you don't add too much liquid to your diet; fruit juice, under the same conditions; an occasional potato or high-protein macaroni or spaghetti; spices; vinegar; non-fattening flavorings and no sugar except saccharin or Sucaryl.

This doesn't mean too much to you? It would, if you studied your food tables. But don't let that bother you! It's all going to be translated into the simplest possible terms for you—so you can't make a mistake—on the very next pages. Now I'm just taking you behind the scenes, so you'll understand what your diet is all about, as you think yourself thin.

CHAPTER 20

Mind over platter

HERE IS WHAT YOU MAY EAT—and feel fine, and full— and still lose weight satisfactorily. Be well fed and get slender at the same time. Sound impossible? Not if you've gone along with me all the way, up to now.

In the morning, after you've "wrung yourself out," please weigh yourself—and mark down your weight. You should do this every day!

Then drink one glass of water. You may put half a lemon in it, or two teaspoonfuls of cider vinegar—if your doctor says that you may. Good for you, some say. But certainly not a necessity.

Then take your exercises—at least ten minutes of them. Take a hot bath, followed by a cold shower— both hot and cold can be showers, if you prefer. I prefer. Then give yourself a brisk rub-down with a rough Turkish towel— so that your blood really tingles, if the exercises and the hot and cold bath didn't do it.

Rub oil or cream on your face and, if you're feminine, apply careful make-up. If you're a man, the same routine— even to oil on the face—but a shave instead of make-up, as if you didn't know.

225

Breakfast, then. And don't think you're helping your reduction regime by omitting breakfast. On the contrary, you're hindering it, for you'll become so hungry you'll eat too much at noon—and eat the wrong things. Anyhow, you probably haven't eaten since fairly early the night before—long enough for the stomach to rest, unless you're on a fast. You need this energy!

And speaking of fasts, they aren't harmful at all—if they aren't too long, and if your physician approves. As a matter of fact, a complete fast of a day or two might be an excellent way to start your new regime— your new life. Or maybe a day or two of fruit juices— just fruit juices—from six to eight glasses, one every hour or two—you don't need any more directions than that. On the fast, you have nothing but water. On the fruit-juice diet, you have only fruit juice—citrus fruit, grape juice, apple juice, pineapple juice—any kinds you prefer. An excellent way to start thinking yourself thin.

You're ready for breakfast. It isn't an exciting meal, certainly, but it should be a real meal. It should include fruit, protein and carbohydrates, up to about 200 calories.

Here are some breakfasts for you:

Grapefruit, 1/2 medium
1 egg, boiled, shirred, "dry fried" or scrambled
1 slice of protein or gluten bread, with Special Cheese
    spread—recipe given
Coffee or tea, with saccharin

1 medium orange
2 slices high-protein bread or toast, with Special
      Cheese and non-sugared apple sauce or jelly Tea or
coffee

1 medium tangerine
1 medium apple, sliced, spread with Special Cream
Coffee or tea

1 medium orange
1 helping cereal—high-protein, non-carbohydrate—
   with sweetener
1/2 glass skimmed milk
Coffee or tea

1/2 grapefruit
Two-egg omelet, "Spanish" or plain
1 small piece dry, high-protein bread or toast
Coffee or tea

1 orange
1 soybean muffin, non-fattening jelly and Special
      Cheese
Coffee or tea

1 tangerine
1 small slice of ham
1 piece of gluten bread or toast
Tea or coffee

1/2 grapefruit
Soy-flour pancakes
Non-fattening imitation maple syrup
Tea or coffee

1 orange
1 piece of bacon, dry
1 "dry fried" egg
Tea or coffee

Fruit breakfast:
1 piece of citrus fruit
Any two other fruits, such as small
    bunch of grapes, one pear and one apple or one
    peach and one plum

1/2 grapefruit
1 glass skimmed milk High-
protein crackers, 2 or 3 Tea or
coffee

You get the idea? I don't want to tell you exactly
what to eat. You aren't a prisoner on rations, you know. You
may eat whatever you want—if it contains the nutrition you
need. And I hope, by now, you've learned enough about
nutrition—about your own needs on this special project—
that you can pick out your own foods. For breakfast you
should have one citrus fruit. That is good for you. The
other items may be chosen by you, and will depend on
what you feel like eating, the sea-

sonable fruits, the weather, etc. In hot weather, you may prefer a crisp, ready-to-eat cereal and cool skimmed milk. In winter, you may want an egg or a bit of bacon or ham. Consult your food lists. Eat at least 200 calories of food at breakfast—preferably fruit and good proteins. Easy? Of course. Citrus fruit at around 50 calories, two other portions of food that average about 75 calories each. Use your brains on your menus. You're thinking yourself thin, you know.

If you have what you like at breakfast—and what passes for a hearty breakfast, these days—you won't be starved, when luncheon time comes. You're to have a hearty luncheon, too. It can be so varied that it is impossible to give you all of the variations. You can eat from 250 to 300 calories—preferably as much protein as possible, together with low-carbohydrate vegetables.

On days when you do not feel like eating meat, you might have:

An omelet or scrambled eggs, and a fresh vegetable salad.

In fact, that is a perfect luncheon—and variations of it may be served over and over again.

Another good luncheon, when you don't want to eat meat, is one consisting of a couple of hot vegetables—low in carbohydrates—and a mixed salad. I'm not going to give you a list of the vegetables you can have, hot or cold. We've gone over that! It's up to you to pick the vegetables that are in season, that you enjoy and feel like eating. They may be eaten with any of the dressings given with the recipes. If you eat out, you can carry salad dressing in a little bottle or use only a little commercial dressing.

A fish luncheon is excellent. This may consist of any hot fish, with a bit of potato, if you like, and a salad. Broiled fish, a small boiled potato and a lettuce and cucumber salad forms a perfect combination—and one I think you'll enjoy. Another excellent seafood luncheon is one consisting of shrimps, crabmeat or lobster, with lettuce, cucumbers and salad dressing.

If you are not on a diet which limits liquids at meals, you may have a small glass of tomato juice before your main course, or a cup of consommé or vegetable soup. I believe, though, that you'll be better off without this extra liquid at luncheon.

Chicken salad—just chicken salad, with a bit of gluten bread or toast—is another fine and well-balanced luncheon, especially if it has generous quantities of chicken, celery and lettuce in it.

Lettuce and tomato salad, with a generous helping of cottage cheese or special diet cheese, is another fine luncheon.

If you eat lunch at drug store counters—and so many people do!—you may find that sandwiches are about all you can get. Then order a sandwich that has a generous filling—preferably one that is served with a lot of lettuce—and do not eat the top piece of bread. With this, you may have tomato juice or fruit juice. This is a well-balanced luncheon.

If you like ice cream, and wish you could eat it on a diet, why not have it for luncheon? Though it is high in calories, containing, as it does, both cream and sugar, as an occasional luncheon it isn't half bad. Neither is a cup of tea and a piece of plain cake.

You may prefer meat at luncheon. If you do, you may have practically any kind of meat, without extra sauce—hamburger, steak, liver, kidneys—almost any meat you can name. With it you may have one potato —and then you have eaten your starchy vegetable allowance, and should not have a starchy vegetable at dinner. If you don't have a potato, you may have a couple of hot low-carbohydrate vegetables—or a mixed salad of any low-carbohydrate vegetables that you feel like eating. Hamburger and an endive salad make a perfect luncheon. So does liver with a bit of bacon, cabbage or string beans. Frankfurters and sauerkraut form another well-balanced, high-protein luncheon. Good, too! Use your brains! Choose the food you enjoy when you enjoy it, providing it is high in protein. Combine it with a low-calorie food. Then you have? a perfect luncheon —one that will satisfy your hunger and carry you through the afternoon. You'll reduce on it, too.

At four or five o'clock, you'll probably want a bite to eat. It's much better to have something then, than to get so hungry that you overeat, when dinner time comes. If you've had a hard day at business—or even at home—a pick-up will give you new energy. This is when you'll take your cocktail—if you feel you need it. You probably will be better off with another sort of pick-up. The English custom of afternoon tea is worth following. Hot tea and a very small sandwich or diet cookie, iced tea with a bite to eat in warm weather, or a glass of milk and a cracker are good. A glass of fruit juice and a cracker or cookie, an apple and a bit of cheese, a pear and cheese, a dish of carrot sticks, or celery stuffed with special cheese mixture and slices of cucumber are also satisfying. You'll find a lot of things you'll like to eat at this time—things that are not fattening, but that are good for you. Because you're eating only a little food, you may have liquids with this meal—the only meals when liquids are allowed on this diet are the light meals such as this between-meal pickup and the bite you have last thing at night.

Dinner is, of course, your important meal of the day. I hope you make rather a ceremony of it. Even if you are dieting and have to omit things that, up to this time, have been important to you, you can still have a fine and nourishing and interesting meal.

Your dinner will depend, of course, on your, pocket-book. What doesn't I I could recommend very luxurious meals that maybe you couldn't afford—and you'd feel that you had to turn to your former fattening meals because of the price. Reduction diets are not inexpensive— but you can find inexpensive items, if you search for them.

You'll want a first course, to make the dinner seem festive. This course may be shrimps, lobster or crab meat—all low in calories and high in protein. But all, unfortunately, expensive. Or, California style, you may like a salad for your first course. This works out very well— for you will enjoy your salad then more than you would after the meat course, when it may have lost its savor, for you are no longer so hungry for it. Your salad will depend, of course, on the season. Any combination of low-carbohydrate vegetables will be good.

Or, for a first course, you may enjoy a simple antipasto or hor d'oeuvres. This could consist of stuffed celery, with special diet cheese filling, perhaps a half of a stuffed egg, a thin slice of salami, some pickled mushrooms, a few artichoke hearts, cooked celery root, pickled beets, sour or dill pickles, radishes, spears of French endive, flowerlets of cauliflower. Not all at one meal, of course! You can use your imagination, and find inexpensive good foods for your first course.

For your main course, you should have meat or fish. Meat, as many days as you can. Fish, on the days when fish is indicated, either because of religion or custom—or expense. Any non-fat fish is excellent. For the meat course, I don't have to make suggestions, Fm sure. Pot roast, meat loaf, hamburgers, frankfurters, kidneys, liver—beef, calves' or pork—sweetbreads, brains, tripe, roast beef, steak—as much steak as you can afford—lamb, veal, fresh ham, boiled or baked ham, turkey, chicken or any other fowl.

With your meat, serve vegetables—one or two will be sufficient. They may be served in fairly large quantities, so they will be filling, if you choose the low-calorie vegetables. Tomatoes and okra, tomatoes and celery, cabbage, brussels sprouts, spinach—look at your lists.

And now I have a surprise for you. A reward for

working hard on your diet. Most reduction diets are woefully lacking in desserts. I can, of course, recommend cheese and crackers or fruit. But I have more than that! How would you like a dessert that tastes like whipped cream, and may be given any flavor, or mixed with fruits? This dessert is my own discovery! I could have sold it to a food company. But I preferred putting it with my recipes—so you'll feel that you're really getting something. I'm giving you a present! You won't want this dessert every day, any more than you'd want whipped cream every day. I worked hard on the recipes for you, but this one came by accident. If I were the type, I'd call it an inspiration. I serve it to company —and my guests think they are getting a rich, high-caloried, forbidden dessert. When you aren't having Think Yourself Thin Magicream for dessert, you'll still want fruit or cheese. The fruit may be practically any fresh fruit, or any canned fruit that is canned without added sugar, or from which the sugar syrup has been washed away. The cheese may be any cheese, but preferably the special diet creams.

You may want a bite to eat before you go to bed at night. A lot of people like to eat then. A glass of skimmed milk—if you haven't had your quota of two glasses for the day—would be fine. You might have a cracker with it, if you haven't used up your bread allowance. An apple with a bit of cheese is a fine midnight snack. Another late-hour bite is a slice of cold meat. Some people have their one after-dinner drink late at night.

Or you may have a glass of fruit juice, if you haven't used up all of your liquid allowance.

Write down what you have eaten during the day. You'll be able to tell in a minute how many calories you have left out of your "allowance." Choose food that fits into these for that last small meal.

This is your daily program for thinking yourself thin. From weighing in, in the morning, to writing down the foods you've eaten at night, and checking them with your food allowance for the day. Five meals! A well-rounded menu of good things to eat. And the kind of exercise you need.

As you begin to lose, I'm sure you'll become optimistic over your diet—over life in general. You'll begin to look better, and feel better, too. You'll look younger—and you'll actually be younger in everything but chronological age—as your better self emerges from its false envelope of fat, and you no longer have to carry an extra burden around with you. As you become slim and erect and firm, you'll face life with a confidence that a fat, flabby person couldn't possibly feel or understand. Let's drink to your health—in a beaker of your calorie-counted skimmed milk or tomato juice !

CHAPTER 21

You eat at home

THIS ISN'T A BOOK of iron-clad menu rules. "Eat liver on Tuesday, followed by meat cakes on Wednesday." How do I know if you feel like eating liver on Tuesday! I resent it when someone tells me what I must or must not do, when there's no reason in the world for it. I don't like people to do my thinking for me when I have a chance to do it for myself, instead. That's why I tell you what you should eat, as far as nutrition is concerned, and then hope you'll plan your own menus. In other words, you'll have to do your own thinking! And eat what you want to eat—within the rules. Think yourself thin!

Now you know what you can eat. Read Chapter 19 over again—and again—if you're in doubt.

BREAKFAST:
    Any citrus fruit
    Egg or protein equivalent
    Tea or coffee with sacharin or Sucaryl
LUNCHEON:
    Meat or its equivalent in high protein
    One or two low-carbohydrate vegetables

TEA:
Tea or fruit drink
High-protein bread, to equal 130 calories, in all.
Or a cocktail—same calories—if you must!

DINNER :
First course to equal about 75 calories
Meat—a hearty portion Vegetables, low
carbohydrates Desserts—from allowed list

NIGHT SNACK:
Same as tea—about 130 calories

DAILY ALLOWANCE :
Two slices of protein bread or high-protein crackers
Two glasses of skimmed milk

If you don't eat your bread allowance at tea or at breakfast, it can be eaten with the other meals. Your milk allowance is up to 2 cups—one pint—of skimmed milk—really skimmed, I mean. This may be distributed as you want to distribute it. With your coffee or tea. As a drink at breakfast or at teatime or at night. Again —it's up to you.

That is a review of your diet. Memorize it! Study your food tables. You'll be able to plan your meals as well as any expert. You are an expert! Consult your doctor when you first plan. Then follow the plan.

After your weight is normal, you might reduce a few pounds more, so you'll have a "reserve" and can gain a pound or two without worrying about it. Maybe, once you're normal, you won't gain! And remember that a small waist line equals a long life line—or so they tell me.

When your weight is just right, you may add a few more foods to your diet, if you like, perhaps larger portions of high-protein foods—and remember that even high-protein foods are fattening, if you eat more than your system needs. You may add a little more bread and butter. I wouldn't add too much starch or sweets, even when you find you can have more calories. Just not good for you. And you want to stay well—and look well and young, I know.

"But I eat at home," you wail. "How can I always eat the right things?"

If you live alone, it's the easiest thing in the world. Just buy the right foods for you! If you're part of a family, it's just as easy, too—if you put your mind to it. You're thinking this out, remember?

At breakfast, you'll have no trouble at all. You omit hot breads, if there are hot breads, and eat fewer eggs, if the family goes in for heavy egg eating. One piece of your special toast, with your special dressing, instead of several slices of buttered toast. As a matter of fact, breakfast will offer few difficulties—the average family doesn't eat much breakfast these days. You may even be eating more than any of the others.

"What do you mean, diet?" the wife of a dieting husband said to me the other day. "George eats more breakfast than I do. We used to have just coffee and toast. Now he's got to have eggs or meat and fruit. I should think he'd get fatter, eating all he does."

"Is he fatter ?" I asked.

"No, curiously enough, he's lost sixteen pounds. I don't understand it."

She'll understand it when she reads this. So will the other non-breakfast eaters, when the dieting member of the family suddenly starts eating more than they do. Breakfast is good for you. It gives you energy for your work. It stimulates your metabolism. It keeps your mind away from food—from being hungry, from thinking about food when you shouldn't be thinking about food.

For luncheon, you won't have at all a difficult time of it. If the family has soup, you omit the soup. Simple as that! Soups may not be fattening—except for cream soups—but they give you too much liquid. Fine for the rest of the family, but not for you. Now the soup manufacturers are shaking their heads! If the family has creamed eggs, have your eggs served without the cream sauce—or with only a trifle of the sauce, for flavor. If they have creamed vegetables, have your vegetables served plain. Skip desserts at lunch time.

For luncheon sandwiches, you must omit part of the bread and all of the butter. And don't eat fattening fillings, such as regulation jellies and peanut butter. You'll find that it isn't too difficult to eat the right things, get enough to eat, and still join a family luncheon.

Dinner isn't difficult either, once you put your mind to it. If you're doing the cooking, you can combine your meals with the family meals, so that everyone is getting enough to eat.

If you're having baked chicken or turkey, you simply omit, for yourself, the dressing, the cranberry sauce— unless you make it especially for you—and most of the potatoes. That will leave you with the turkey and vegetables—an ample main course.

If you serve the family spaghetti or noodles or rice, be sure to have, too, a low-carbohydrate vegetable— and you eat the vegetable which is low in calories. Don't start eating a small portion of macaroni and cheese, or you'll find you've eaten a large portion of it. if you omit everything else but the low-carbohydrate vegetables for the main part of your meal, then you may have spaghetti or macaroni—or any of the high-calorie dishes.

Omit all "fancy" dishes from your own menus. The sauces are out, but when you serve mushrooms, you may have a double share. All hot breads are out—you must be satisfied with a slice of gluten bread. But you can join the family in eating meats, vegetables, fruits without sweet sauces, all of the main courses that are not prepared with too many fattening ingredients. And, if you're doing the cooking, learn to do without those same forbidden foods. You can give your family enough health-giving dishes so that they'll be well and strong— and grow properly, if there are young people in the family—and still be able to choose your own food, so that you'll get enough, too. It's all a matter of putting your mind to it—of becoming a thinking human being. Think yourself into being a sensible manager. Think about the foods for the whole family, so that everyone will be well and sensibly nourished. Think yourself thin!

Some of your special gourmet dishes may be out entirely. Others will be reserved for special occasions. If you learn to use flavorings and seasonings, you can gain a reputation for being a fine cook, without using too many fattening ingredients.

When you have company, serve a company dinner—and give yourself just what you should eat. You'll be surprised how no one notices that you aren't eating a lot of everything ! If your dinner is good enough, your guests will be too busy devouring their own portions. And curiously enough, you'll take a peculiar sort of delight in serving rich foods that you can't eat yourself.

Of course it won't do a bit of harm to give your guests diet foods. A lot of them may be overweight, anyhow. And if they aren't, a single fattening dish will balance the dinner, so that they'll get enough fat and feel well fed. Yorkshire pudding and baked potatoes added to the roast means that you can eat everything else—the first course of mixed hors d'oeuvres, the meat, the vegetables, the fruit dessert.

The wisest thing to do is to choose your own meal first. This isn't selfish—it means that the others, whether guests or family, will get high-protein and good vegetables. Then add one or two "forbidden" foods to the list, and bread and butter, to make a more rounded meal for the others. And then, at dinner time, you can get a good meal and eat everything but the added high-calorie dishes, and the others will be well—even generously—fed. Simplest thing in the world, once you think about it.

What about those special foods that you can buy for yourself—and that the rest of the family may like, too? The health-food stores are full of hundreds of articles that are supposedly low in calories and high in proteins. The trouble is that a lot of them are tasteless, too. I've done a lot of shopping and discovering. I've asked a lot of questions. Here are some of the foods I like. You can try them, and if you like them, add them to your meals. If you don't like them, just never order them again. Simple, isn't it? These are all foods made by manufacturers who cater to folks on diets. As I'm not being paid by any of them, and have no interests in any of the companies (I wish I had!), I'm just picking out a few that seem satisfactory to me. You can make your own discoveries—and you'll find new ones every day, I'm sure.

My "staff of life," instead of ordinary breads, consists of low-calorie products, which may not taste nearly as good as hot, Southern corn bread or muffins, slathered with fresh country butter, but which serve very well for a substitute.

I like, very much, the products made by Anthony Alphonse de Bole. His address is 120 Sullivan Street, New York. Mr. de Bole manufactures artichoke foods that are quite low in carbohydrates. I especially like his artichoke toast, which is salt-free, and comes in large five-dollar boxes. B. Altman, as well as a lot of the health stores and department stores, also carries Mr.

de Bole's products in smaller boxes. He makes a good bread stick, a rather sweet rusk, flavored with anise, and excellent low-carbohydrate noodles, both plain and with spinach. I use the artichoke toast daily—the best recommendation I can give it. Each piece is said to average 10 calories. The crumbs from the toast or the bread-sticks are excellent to use in fruit puddings and for "breading," a delicacy usually forbidden those on a diet. They may be used, too, in filling green peppers and in meat loaves.

The Dietetic Food Company, at 5228 New Utrecht Avenue, Brooklyn, New York, has excellent foods for folks on diets. A young lady named Miss G. Binstock takes care of my orders—you might write to her—or buy the Dietetic foods at department or health stores. I like best, of all their products, their "Special Dietetic Crackers." These are salt-free and have a delicious flavor. They are made of gluten, soy bean and wheat flours, have a 40% protein and a 23% carbohydrate content, and average 13 calories per cracker. They, and their toast and bread sticks, are excellent with milk or cheese spreads, or at any meal.

This same company makes a good gluten toast, chocolate syrups, cookies. For sweets, they make a chocolate-flavored miniature bonbon, with fruit and nuts, that averages 21 calories, against 100 calories for an ordinary sweet. Their candy jellies—very well flavored little gum drops—contain only about 5 calories each, and are sugar-free. Under the trade name of Dia-mel, they have dozens of other excellent products.

The Charles Kilgore Company, in Yonkers, New York, manufactures the Dietician Brand of low-calorie foods. Some of these are very good, and you might experiment with them. I prefer their Assorted Chocolates Substitute, which contain about half the calories of regulation chocolates. They manufacture a lot of other things, too.

The Battle Creek Food Company, of Battle Creek, Michigan, is one of the best known health-food companies in America. They manufacture many excellent low-calorie, high-protein foods. I liked best their canned gluten bread, which is soft and moist—and will stay that way, if you keep it in the can in the refrigerator. They make an excellent soy gluten wafer, fine with nearly everything, that has a 49% protein, 15% fat and 13% carbohydrate content. Each wafer has a 12-calorie food value·

The Kellogg Company is putting out a fine new wheat-germ product—flaked wheat germ, that tastes like any good breakfast food, but contains all of the good nutriments of wheat germ, which, as you know, is a valuable food, full of vitamins and fairly high in protein, though three ounces give about 400 calories of food value.

The Chicago Dietetic Supply House, at 1750 West Van Bur en Street, Chicago 12, Illinois, manufactures a full line of low-calorie foods, under the Cellu Brand. These can be bought at most of the health-food stores. This is a most comprehensive list of foods—and you'll probably find some you'll like a great deal.

The Loeb Dietetic Food Company, New York 33, is

one of the best known diet-food companies in America. They manufacture dozens of good products. I like best their aerated bread and rolls, which remain fresh for months, are salt-free and are a fine base for any spreads or just as a bread substitute. Their cookies and puddings are good, too.

The Isrin-Oliver Company, at 169 Spring Street, New York 12, manufactures a number of gourmet foods— but has a number of foods on its list for those who are trying to lose or maintain weight, too. They make a good griddle-cake mixture, which can also be used for thickening, a nice imitation maple syrup, and a good salt substitute, with a pleasing flavor of its own, called Fortissimo Seasoning.

The Utt Juice Company, of Tustin, California, has a whole series of pure fruit juices, without added sugar. They are fine as drinks, when sweetened with your favorite sugar substitute, and properly diluted. With unsweetened gelatin added, they make good desserts, too. I prefer their red raspberry juice. Welch's grape juice, unsweetened, as well as the unsweetened fruit juice of all reputable companies, makes fine desserts when sweetened and thickened.

The Lord Calvert Beverage Company of Brooklyn, New York, manufactures low-calorie dietetic carbonated beverages that contain about 8 calories per eight-ounce glass. Sweetened with sorbitol and saccharin, these come in cola, cream soda, grape, raspberry and ginger ale flavors. The Berry Springs Mineral Water Company of Pawtuckct, Rhode Island, makes excellent beverages, too.

Nearly all of these companies put up fruits, either water-packed or without added sugar. All of them are satisfactory. Among the best, according to my tastes, are those in the Special Dietetic Pack of the Richmond-Chase Company of San Jose, California. They call these products "Diet-Delight." Your neighborhood shop can get them for you, I know. Sweeten the juice with Sucaryl, and the result is as good as any canned fruit I've ever tasted. The Dole Company, well known for its unsweetened pineapple juice—a favorite with all dieters—also puts up non-sweetened sliced pineapple—a valuable addition to any reduction diet.

The Ditex Company of Chicago puts up excellent foods. I like especially their small cans of well-seasoned fruits without sugar. The Pratt-Low Company of Santa Clara, California, puts up excellent fruits, also, which are perfect for the dieter.

A number of the companies I've mentioned manufacture high-protein spaghetti and macaroni. Ask for them, and don't eat any of these starch products unless they are high in protein. One that I like best is made by the Buitoni Company, with factories in Jersey City, New York, France and Italy. Your shop can get these for you, I know. Buitoni makes spaghetti, macaroni, and perciatelli which has a 20 per cent as well as a 35 per cent protein content, with a comparatively low amount of carbohydrates. The box gives the percentages of the amino acids and the vitamins, showing that they are excellent in food values. You'll be able to eat many ordinarily forbidden dishes with these high-protein products.

Like tuna fish? Usually it is very high in calories. Now the Van Camp Sea Food Company, of Terminal Island, California, has decided to come to the help of dieters, and has put out a special Chicken of the Sea product. This is called their Dietetic Pack. It is low in sodium and in fat, and very high in protein. An excellent addition to the dieter's list of food.

I haven't even thought it necessary to mention every dieter's standby—Knox's Gelatin. You probably have been using it for years, anyhow. Practically pure protein, it is ideal in every way—it is not only good in itself, but it enables you to make lovely dishes that, otherwise, wouldn't be available. As a lot of my special recipes contain gelatin—and I always use Knox's, because of its convenient pack and quick-dissolving properties—I need not say any more about it here. It's super! I don't see how anyone on a diet could keep house and serve foods that have variety and interest without it. Ordinary gelatin dessert powders are full of sugar, you know.

Many of the dietetic food companies package their own gelatin powders, sweetened with saccharin or other non-sugar sweetners and pleasantly flavored, and you may enjoy those, too, but gelatin can be your real standby, both for desserts and main-course dishes.

The Diet-Rite Company of New York, one of the new companies interested in diet foods, is making several very good products. They make a tiny cracker, good for that extra-meal snack, that is excellent in flavor. It is called "Slim Treet." Their "Slim Tays-Tees" are good little cookies, averaging nine calories.

Of course, nearly all canned vegetables are satisfactory for diets. For an unusual vegetable, you might try Hearts of Palms, of the Kanana Brand. Hearts of artichokes are a valuable addition to salads, too.

Canned fruits, unless they are diet-packed—water or fruit juice, and no added sugar—are not good for you. If you must use them, pour off the syrup—you can use it for the non-dieting members of your family—rinse off the fruit with water, add some non-sugar sweetening, and serve nearly dry.

Of course, lean meats, fresh vegetables and fruits and pot cheese, together with skimmed milk and buttermilk, are your best bets, together with a reasonable amount of these diet foods. You can eat these—and eat alone, or with your family—and be well fed—and so can they, now that you know what to eat, yourself—and what to add to your diet, so that your family and guests may dine well, too. It isn't so bad, being on a reduction diet It may even be fun !

CHAPTER 22

You eat out

MANY OF YOU are going to pounce on me now. I can just hear you. I have heard you.

"It's all very well to diet, when you're at home. But what about when you eat out? I'm just fine at home—but when I go out I throw all discretion to the wind and eat everything, and gain back all I've lost for the week."

I know what you mean! I've been through that, too. You've got to do a mental job on yourself. Not so much steel yourself against eating the wrong things as to accept, calmly, the fact that you can't eat everything. Don't fight against the wrong things! That's too much of a defeatist attitude. Just tell yourself, "Those things are not for me. I may as well face it now as any other time. I'm living a new life—and the new life happens to exclude everything that isn't good for me."

It may take you a while to accept the right idea—to have your subconscious accept it. Once you do, and all's well, you'll gain a sort of aloof, almost superior attitude, and almost enjoy not eating the things that are wrong for you. I can pass a bake shop or a candy shop full of goodies and stare at them without even thinking that I might buy and eat them. Of course I'd like them. But there are other things I'd like, too—a new mink coat, to be eighteen and beautiful, to have a million dollars, to see the world in a state of sanity. I can't have any of these—including the goodies. So I accept things as they are, and enjoy the things I have, instead. It may sound a bit on the corny side, but accept things as they are—and count your blessings. You'll be surprised to find how many you have—even if eating unlimited quantities of fattening foods isn't one of them. Other people . . . Other people . . . Oh, well—other people I

The chief difficulty in dining out is the before-meal nibble—bread and butter. There they are—on the table before any other food is served—and for free, too. Easy to eat—and ruination to a strict reduction diet. Leave them alone! And don't eat the delicious hot breads that will probably be passed to you during the meal. One slice of bread should be your bread allowance when dining out.

You won't have any trouble with breakfast. From the best restaurant in town to the least expensive lunch counter, there will be just the things for you. Citrus fruit, coffee or tea without sugar, to be sweetened with your own saccharin or Sucaryl. One egg and a slice of unbuttered whole wheat bread—if your high-protein bread isn't available—or two eggs and no bread at all, or a slice of ham—no fat—and one slice of bread. You'll make out.

Your lunches can be simplified, too. In a "best" restaurant, you can have liver and bacon and a green vegetable, or a very good salad, with shrimp, lobster or chicken, or even a small steak and a mixed green salad. No one will care at all that you don't order dessert—though you can always have half a grapefruit or a piece of melon, if that helps out the luncheon.

Your dinners won't be too difficult if you don't stimulate your appetite and weaken your will power with alcohol. At the Plaza Hotel in New York—one of the smartest hotels in the world—they cater to people on diets—they get the conservative older crowd, for the most part. They'll bring you skimmed milk, if you ask for it. And they make a special salad, with their Diet Dressing, which is made with a mineral oil base. Very good, too. You won't have any trouble there. With a shrimp or oyster cocktail to start the meal, a mixed grill, a salad, a glass of milk and perhaps a melon or a fruit compote, you've dined very well.

The Colony, as you probably know, is one of New York's most exclusive restaurants. I live practically across the street from it—but it must be the widest street in the world, for too seldom do my escorts suggest that we could just go across the street to dine. And they'd save taxi fare, too! Which really isn't being fair. I've had some delicious meals there—and since I've been dieting, too. The Colony has planned a special diet for its regular diners who want to lose weight. It seems to me it's a bit severe, but I shall give it to you. You may want to follow it in toto, and pretend you're eating the way chic New Yorkers do when they're desperate about getting too fat. You understand enough about diets to sec how low in calories it is—but if it's good enough for Colony patrons, surely it ought to satisfy you. It includes no drinks of any kind—and no extra nibbles between meals. Just three meals a day I Breakfast is always the same—and very meager it is, too. It consists of half a grapefruit, black coffee with saccharin and warm skimmed milk. Less than your special diet, but all you get if you're dieting on the Colony's rules.

The Colony diet was given to me by Helen Bennett, who does publicity for the Colony. She tells me a lot of the dieting patrons use it regularly, too. It has been printed in the book by lies Brody, *The Colony,* published by Greenberg.

Here are your Colony menus for their four-day reduction diet:

First Day

LUNCH: Two lamb chops; one raw tomato.

DINNER: Minute steak; lettuce salad with mineral oil dressing; tea and lemon with saccharin if desired.

Second Day

LUNCH: Two broiled lamb chops; two raw tomatoes; one sliced orange; tea with lemon and saccharin.

DINNER: Half a grapefruit; half broiled chicken; stewed tomatoes; cooked spinach with a hard-boiled egg; tea with lemon and saccharin.

Third Day

> LUNCH: Orange juice; two scrambled eggs made with water instead of cream; stewed tomatoes; one slice of Melba toast with jelly; tea with lemon and saccharin.
>
> DINNER: Half a grapefruit; broiled minute steak; lettuce and tomato salad with mineral oil dressing; coffee with saccharin.

Fourth Day

> LUNCH: Two broiled lamb chops; cooked carrots; cooked spinach; stewed tomatoes; orange and grapefruit salad with mineral oil dressing; one slice of Melba toast with jelly; tea with saccharin and lemon.
>
> DINNER: Half a grapefruit; broiled minute steak; lettuce and tomato salad with mineral oil dressing; tea with saccharin and lemon.

From El Borracho come menus for these diet dinners:

(1.) Tomato juice or fruit juice; 2 lamb chops; string beans; apple or pear; glass of skimmed milk or tea with lemon and saccharin or black coffee.

(2.) Half grapefruit; lean steak; lima beans or spinach; tomato and avocado salad—very little dressing; skimmed milk; tea or coffee without cream; saccharin.

The figure of the owner, author of *Love and Dishes*¡ Nicky Quattrococchi, speaks well for this diet.

If you eat in what New Yorkers refer to as a "private home"—1 loathe the expression—you'll not fare too well—but you'd undoubtedly eat more than you would if you were eating at the Colony and following their printed diet. You may have to accept a soup—even if it isn't on your diet—if it is served as a first course. But you can avoid gravies and sauces and potatoes and bread and butter—which will probably mean that you can have meat and a vegetable. You'll just have to wave a reluctant hand at your serving of dessert and say, as gracefully as you can:

"That looks wonderful! I'd love to have it! But I must keep on my diet, you know!"

If you sound firm enough—and reluctant enough—you'll make the hostess or host believe that you're practically broken hearted, but that your diet is too important to be broken for anyone. You'll get enough to eat! If not, you can always have that snack when you get home.

Of course, even if you're dining at the Colony, or any other good restaurant, you needn't adhere to the Colony's strict diet. You can chose far more interesting foods, and not add too many calories to your count for the day.

Last night I dined in the Cotillion Room at the Pierre. I had orange juice, while my escort had a cocktail. I had a shrimp cocktail, then, followed by sweetbreads and broccoli with Hollandaise sauce. I took a small helping of the Hollandaise, and my escort finished it up—put it on his peas! Said it tasted good, too. He had a rich concoction of turkey, with a sauce that contained cream and eggs and cheese. It didn't even tempt me. I took a small portion home to Lord Calvert, my Pomeranian. He loved it I But then he liked the bit of my sweetbreads he ate, too. I carry a small plastic box in my bag and take home nibbles for his dinner. I'm glad he isn't a St. Bernard or I could never feed him from restaurant tables. For dessert I had a very nice slice of melon, and didn't even envy the people eating parfaits all around me.

New York's famous Waldorf Astoria always has on its menus excellent food for folks who are dieting.

But don't think you have to eat in an expensive restaurant in order to get good diet food! Night before last I ate at the Automat—the least expensive place to eat in New York. My escorts all seem to be very rich men, who have arrived, or very poor ones who are, I hope, on the way up. I don't know any middle-of-the-road ones, it seems. Maybe there aren't any around! The Automat food is excellent. It is purchased from the same markets that sell to the most expensive restaurants. I'm sure that the conditions are the same in every city— you can find good food at any price you can pay. At the Automat I had, as a first course, a tomato aspic with cottage cheese—very good, too. And I followed this with chopped sirloin steak, kale and turnips—two vegetables I like a lot. The Automat vegetables are especially good—better than in a lot of expensive places, and more varieties to choose from, too. For dessert I had

stewed pears, and because I'm on a' maintenance diet— I
don't have to lose any more, for I weigh no and I'm 5
feet 1 inch—I could eat the syrup, which wasn't very sweet,
anyhow.

Most restaurants do not have special diets. But in
every one you can find food that is right for you. At Mr.
Billingsley's Stork Club, probably New York's best
known restaurant, you can dine on the richest food
obtainable anywhere, or you can eat sensible diet food— and
lose weight, even while you're faring well. At
Schrafft's, which is noted for its excellent food, you can
dine well and not too expensively, and in spite of the fact
that Schrafft's is famous for cakes and candies, you can find
a lot of not too fattening things on their menus, too.
Child's chain of restaurants is as inexpensive as you'll
find, with nice surroundings and good service, in New
York. I dined at all three restaurants—and very well,
too—and found that there were several combinations of
food to form excellent dinners in all three places: New
York's smart Stork Club; the moderately priced Schrafft's;
and the inexpensive—for today—Child's. So here are all
three menus for you, with dinners marked on each one—as
suggestions for what you can eat, when you're dining out.
The prices are those prevailing in September, 1951, and all
of them are a la carte. Child's and Schrafft's also serve
many of these items on special "Club Dinners," which
include an appetizer, entree and vegetables, salad, dessert
and coffee, at prizes ranging from $1.20 to $1.75 and
$1.55 to $2.30, respectively.

Outside of New York, the food is usually less expensive. But wherever you are, you can dine out with comfort and have good meals at practically any restaurant— and still use your brains about choosing non-fattening foods. I don't know all of the states, but those I've been in have all had possibilities for diet, even if you had to miss good things to eat. It's possible to diet very easily in Hollywood, because the movie people are very diet conscious. But I'd say it could be done no matter where you are. There is, for example, no better food any place than in my home state, Arkansas. Yet even there, you can dine at the Marion or the Sam Peck in Little Rock; at the Majestic in Hot Springs; at the Goldman in Fort Smith—my home town—or at the Basin Park or Crescent Hotel in Eureka Springs, and eat exceedingly well, even if you have to omit fried chicken with cream gravy and hot biscuits, two of the state's specialties.

On the following menus, the foods which you can eat while dieting are indicated in regular type, and the fattening foods which you should *not* order are in italics. But of course you know these yourself, by now, because you've been studying your food charts! When a dish that is allowed is served with a fattening gravy or fried potatoes, just ask your waiter to omit it or substitute another lower-calorie item. You don't have to be afraid to speak up. Most restaurants are only too happy to oblige the dieter.

CHILDS

APPETIZERS

Fresh Vegetable Soup .15   *Chicken Rice Soup* .15
Tomato Juice   .15   Chilled Pineapple Juice .15

ENTREES

Roast Tom Turkey, *Dressing, Gravy, Cranberry Sauce, Candied Sweet Potato,* Green Peas 1.30
Choice Tenderloin Steak, *French Fried Potatoes,* Fresh Vegetable, Chefs Salad *with Russian Dressing* 2,25
Deep Fried Sea Scallops, Sauce Tartare, Whipped Potatoes and Garden Spinach 95
Braised Beef and Mushrooms *with Gravy,* Whipped Potatoes, Green Peas 90
Chopped Sirloin Grill, *French Fried Potatoes,* Green Peas .. 1.05
Breaded Cutlet of Milkfed Veal, Tomato Sauce, French Fried Potatoes, Lima Beans 1.05
Baked Sugar Cured Ham with Red Cherry Sauce, Candied Sweet Potato, Buttered Lima Beans 1.05
Broiled Halibut Steak *with Parsley Butter Sauce, French Fried Potatoes,* Garden Spinach... 1.15

SALADS AND SANDWICHES

Salad Bowl—Julienne Turkey and Baked Ham tossed with Fresh Pineapple and Garden Greens... 90
Hot Brisket Corned Beef Sandwich, *served with French Fried Potatoes* and Pickle Chips 75
Sandwich Plate-Sliced Ham, Chopped Egg and Ripe Tomato Slices *on three slices of Buttered Toast* 65

Freshly Baked Rolls or Muffins

DESSERTS

French Vanilla, Chocolate,
  Strawberry or Coffee Ice
  Cream   .20
Creamy Rice Pudding   .15
Nesselrode Layer Cake   .15
Seedless Half Grape
  fruit   .20
Jello with Whipped
  Cream   .15
Green Apple Pie   .15
  a la Mode   .25

Special Strawberry Sundae,
  Whipped Cream   .30
Chocolate Marshmallow
  Nut Sundae   .40
Banana Split   .50
Cocoanut Custard Pie   .20
Fresh Fruit Cup   .20
Blue Cheese with
  Toasted Crackers   .30
Pineapple Royale
  Sundae   .45

BEVERAGES

Tea or Coffee   .10

SCHRAFFT'S

APPETIZERS

Supreme of Pineapple		Chilled Vegetable Juice	
and Oranges	.30	Cocktail	.20
Cream of Tomato Soup	.25	*Chicken Consommé*	.25

ENTREES

Schrafft's Fresh Vegetable Dinner—*Candied Sweet Potato,* Grilled
  Tomato Creole, Cauliflower *an Gratin,* Carrots and Peas, Fresh
  String Beans and Broiled Fresh Mushrooms *on Toast*   1.00 Roast
Prime Ribs of Beef *with Lyonnaise Potatoes* and Cauliflower
  au Gratin   2.00
Minute Steak *with Hashed Brown Potatoes*   3.50 Roast Leg of
Lamb *with Currant Jelly,* Mashed Potatoes *and
  Glazed Beets*   1.50
Broiled Chicken (half) *with Candied Sweet Potatoes* and Fresh
  String Beans Julienne   1.70 *Noodles with Ham in Fricassee
Sauce, Glazed Pineapple Ring
  with Banana and French Fried Eggplant*   .95
Chicken Pot Pie with New Vegetables and Potato Cover   .95
*Fried Oysters with Sauce Tartare and Hashed Brown
  Potatoes*   1.25

SALADS AND SANDWICHES

Salad *Bowl—Avocado Pear,* Apple, Tomato and Mixed Greeni
  with Grated American Cheese and Currant Muffins   .95
Tomato Stuffed with Chopped Chicken and Celery Salad   .95
Club Sandwich-Sliced Breast of Turkey, Bacon and Tomato *on
Toast, with Mayonnaise*   .95

Assorted Hot Breads

DESSERTS AND FRUITS

Apple Delight with
   Foamy Sauce   .25
Ice Cream Cake with
   Hot Butterscotch
   Sauce and Ahnonds .35
Custard Fhating IsL·nd
   *With Whipped Cream.*25
Stewed Calimyrna Figs .20

Supreme of Pineapple
   and Oranges   .30
Old-Fashioned Jelly
   Cake .25-a *la Mode*   .40
Chocolate Cream Pie   .30
Apple Fie   .25
Danish Pastry   .15-.20
Broadway Sundae   .80

ICE CREAMS

Strawberry Ice Cream .20
Coffee Ice Cream   .20
Assorted Ice Creams-Vanilla,
Chocolate, Coffee,
Strawberry   .35
Chocolate Mint
   Ice Cream Soda   .30
Cherry Marshmallow
   Sundae   .30

Vanilla Ice Cream   .20
Chocolate Ice Cream   .20
Hot Butterscotch Sundae .30
Crushed Pineapple
   Ice Cream Soda   .30
Crushed Strawberry
   Ice Cream Soda   .30

BEVERAGES

Schrafft's Orange Pekoe
   Tea-Pot   .20
Schrafft's Special Blend
   Coffee-Cup   .15
Schrafft's Luxuro Hot
   Chocolate with
   Whipped Cream   .20

Sanka—Cup   .15
Milk   .15
Buttermilk   .15

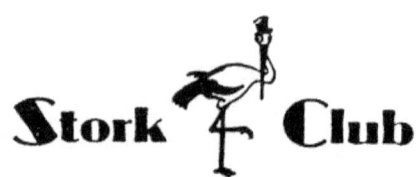

Stork Club

OYSTERS, CLAMS AND COCKTAILS

Blue Point Oysters   1.00
Little Neck Clams   .85
Clams Rockefeller   2.00
Tomato Juice Cocktail   .75
Lobster Cocktail   2.25 Clam
Juice Cocktail   1.00

Cape Cod Oysters   1.25
Clam Stew   2.00
Cherrystone Clams   .95
Crab Meat Cocktail   2.00
Shrimp Cocktail   1.85

APPETIZERS

*Hors D'Oeuvres
Parisienne* 2.25 Stuffed
Celery   1.50 *Canape of
Anchovies*   1.50 Smoked
Sturgeon   2.25 *Nova Scotia
Salmon*   2.00 Fresh Fruits
Supreme,
Maraschino   1.25

Terrine de Foie Gras   4.00
Crab Ravigotte   2.25 *Crab
Meat Suzette*   2.25 Tomato
Surprise   1.50 Virginia Ham
2.25

SOUPS

Chicken Broth   .85 *Onion
Soup Gratine*   1.10
Consomme Printaniere   1.00
*Petite Marmite
Henri IV*   1.25
Chicken Okra   .90

Boula· au Gratin   1.10
Cream of Tomato   .90
Consomme Bellevue   .90
Puree St. Germain   .85
*Clear Green Turtle aux
Xeres*   1.40

EGGS

Scrambled Eggs *with*
  Sausage or Bacon 2.00
Chicken Livers 2.50
Omelette Espagnole 2.25
Poached Eggs
  on toast 2.00
Poached Eggs
  a la Reine 2.25
Shirred Eggs
  Portugaise 2.25

Eggs Benedict 2.50
Gachot Smithfield Virginia
  Ham and Eggs 2.25
Plain Omelette 2.00
Waffles and Sausages 2.25
Fried Eggs, French Style,
  with Ham 2.50

ENTREES

Tournedos Saute, Jacqueline 5.50
Roast Prime Ribs of Beef 4.25
Minced Chicken, Madras 3.75
Smothered Chicken, *Southern Style* 4.00
Steak Minute, Steve Hannagan 5.00
Breaded Veal Cutlet, Marechale 3.75
Broiled Lamb Chops, Nicoise 4.00
Chicken a L· King 3.75
Breast of Guinea Hen, Shermane 4.25
Sliced Capon, Asparagus Tips, Mornay 3.75
Veal Chop, Barbara 4.25
Chicken Hamburger, Walter Winchell 4.00
Creamed Chicken Hash, Marie Rose 4.00
Broiled Breast of Chicken, Morton Downey 4.25
Broiled Sweetbread, Virginia 3.50
Broiled Tenderloin of Beef, Mushrooms 5.50
Calf's Liver Saute, *French Fried Onions* 3.75
Broiled Sirloin Steak (for one), Mushrooms 6.00
Noisette Lamb, Sortilege 4.25

FISH

Broiled Filet of Sole, St. Germain   3.75
Shrimps a l·Indienne, Rice   3.25
Crab Meat Dewey   3.50
Lobster Cardinal   4.00
Brook Trout Saute, Doria   3.50
Deviled Lobster   3.50
Stuffed Deviled Crab   3.00
Frog Legs Provencale   4.00
Lobster Newburg   4.00
Whole Broiled Lobster, *Allumette Potato*
(according to size)

COLD DISHES

Sliced Chicken, Waldorf Salad   3.50
Assorted Cold Cuts, Salade Russe   3.75
Cold Half Lobster, Parisienne   3.75
Sliced Cold Tongue, Chefs Salad   2.75
Steak Tartare   4.25 Cold Roast
Prime Rib of Beef, *Potato Salad*   3.75
Cold Roast Ham, Macedoine Salad   3.00
Catskill Mountain Smoked Turkey, Stork Salad   3.75

SALADS

Chicken and Pineapple
  a la Stork   3.25
Lobster   3.75
Romaine and Lettuce   1.15
Chiffonade   1.50 Shrimp
3.50 Combination   1.50

Crab Meat   3.50
Half Alligator Pear,
  Chicken   3.00
Romaine and
  Grapefruit   1.50
Fruit   2.00 Sunset
2.75 Chefs   2.75

LEGUMES

Broiled Tomato   .75 Egg
Plant, Provencale   1.50
Lima Beans   .90   i0
Braised Celery   1.25
Stewed Fresh
Tomatoes   1.00
  Succotash .90
String Beans and Lima
  Beans   1.00
  Peas   .85

Barbara B. B. 3-in-1   1.50
Hearts of Palm, au
  Gratin   1.50
Brussels Sprouts   1.25 Plain
Spinach .85
Creamed Spinach   1.00
Fried Eggplant   1.00
Broccoli   1.50
Corn Saute, Mexicaine   .85

POMMES

French Fried .75
Saute .75

Souffle .90

Hashed Brown or
  Parisienne .75
Boiled   .65 New
Bermuda   1.00
Delmonico .75
Candied Sweet

Julienne .75
Allumette .75
Au Gratin   1.00
Lyonnaise   1.00
Mashed .75
Baked .75
Fried Sweet
Potatoes   1.00

RAREBITS

Long Island   1.75
Scotch Woodcock   1.85
Yorkshire Buck   1.85

Golden Buck   1.85
Welsh Rarebit   1.50

Bread and Butter   1.00

266
DESSERTS

Apple Pie 1.00
Crepes Maison 2.00
Crepes Suzette 3.00
Coupe aux Marrons 1.75
Baked Alaska
  (for two) 4.00
French Pastry 1.00

Custard Pie 1.00
Peach Melba 1.85
Pear Cardinal 1.75
Souffle Arlequin
  (for two) 3.50
Omelette Souffle 1.80
Coupe Nesselrode 1.75

ICE CREAM AND WATER ICE

Vanilla, Chocolate,
  Strawberry or Coffee .85
Roulade Stork 1.75
Spumoni .90

Coffee Parfait 1.25
Raspberry or Orange
  Ice .85
Eggnog, Maison 1.50

CHEESE

Roquefort, Camembert,
  Stilton, Imported Swiss
  or Petite Gruyere .85
Gold-N-Rich .75
Bel Paese 1.00

Brie .85
American .75
Cream Cheese *with*
  Bar-le-Duc 1.00

COFFEE, TEA, Etc.

Coffee *with Cream* .65
Sanka .65
Hot Chocolate or
  Cocoa 1.25
Cafe Rico 1.25

Demi Tasse .50
Tea .50
Postum .65
Milk .45

CHAPTER 23

Exercise and how to avoid it

You CAN SEE HOW I've been avoiding the subject of exercise. Just the way most overweight folks avoid exercise. Well, here we are! And the truth is that you've got to think yourself into a certain amount of exercise. A very small amount, I assure you. If you think about it in the right way you can practically avoid it—and it will be nearly painless. It's a very important part of thinking yourself thin.

Personally, I loathe all sports. I even loathe being a spectator at sports. One time I was about to purchase a pair of shoes and found they were marked Spectator sport," so I didn't buy them. What if they had been magic shoes, and marched me into the grandstand at a Forest Hills tennis game, or out to the Stadium to the baseball bleachers. A narrow escape, I call it. I still give a sigh of relief when I think of it.

But I know, as well as you do, that the ideal form of exercise is an outdoor one. Baseball, golf, tennis, badminton, skiing, hiking, swimming, rowing—they're all wonderful for you! Next best are the indoor sports: basketball, bowling, gymnasium workouts. If you like them, please take as much of them as you can. You couldn't be doing better for yourself! Even mowing the lawn and shoveling snow are fine exercises. You breath deeply of fresh air. Your system is stimulated, your muscles hardened. I couldn't stand any of them, myself. In fact, though I love life, I think I'd rather be dead than have to do much of any of them. Maybe you feel the same way. I hope you don't. If you like outdoor or indoor exercise, your exercise problem is solved. All you have to do is' to go in a bit strenuously for the sport you like best, and that's that. You don't even have to read the rest of this chapter, except to gloat.

I've discovered, though, that most people who weigh too much hate exercise as much as I do. And exercise seems to hate them back. Fat folks who exercise are seemingly always getting into trouble. They are accident prone. They break legs the first day they try to ski. A baseball hits them in the eye. Or they overdo and have an awful time. Most of them solve the problem by never exercising at all. It's a chicken-and-egg proposition: Do people get fat because they don't exercise, or don't they exercise because they're fat.

Well, anyhow, exercise, per se, won't reduce you Not unless you go all out for it—a sort of eight-hours-a-day health farm training—and even then only because you'll probably be put on a high-protein, nearly all-meat diet. For exercise, among other things, makes you hungry, and unless you're under supervision—your own or a professional's, you'll eat on far more fat than you exercised off.

You've heard, I'm sure, all of the tall tales about how

much you'd have to exercise in order to lose weight. Unfortunately, most of them are true I Maybe it's fortunate —for the overweight. He won't start in on strenuous exercise, knowing it won't do much good for him. For example, you may climb a mountain all day long—and in the ice and snow, too, which takes even more energy— go back to camp, eat a hearty meal—and find you haven't lost any weight at all. If you dieted, you may have lost a pound. Is it worth it? You can walk—not up a mountain, but just in a comparatively straight line, and at a good pace—and lose. That is, if you walk about thirty-four miles you can lose a pound—or two miles to the ounce. Eat one small extra chocolate and you've eaten the mile back again. Of course, you may be a lot firmer, and that will make you look better. Or you may be just tired.

Certainly, regular walking every day is fine for you. Splendid exercise, in fact. But, if you want to reduce at the same time, you must diet, along with the walking. Then you'll really accomplish something.

Like to dance? You may dance—ball room dancing, that is—for half an hour, and lose three hundred calories. Drink two highballs during the evening—or have a couple of orange drinks and a few "nibbles"—and you've eaten it all back again.

Dancing and horseback riding aren't really exercise— not obnoxious ones, anyhow. But if you like those—or any others—do indulge in them, if your doctor thinks you should. But please use the high-protein diet at the same time! Then you'll get in fit condition, and become slender and firm.

Perhaps you'll like less strenuous exercises. You may even experiment with the so-called "passive" exercises. There are a lot of them around. Alas, most of them are rather useless. If you use one for a full hour a day, or longer, it may help you a little. But who has time for that? These passive exercises consist of electric machines, couches with motors which cause light or heavy vibrations, or roller machines. The roller machines are certainly the best. They won't hurt you. They may give you some psychological help. If you use them enough, along with your diet, they may even give you actual help in firming and stimulating you.

If you like mechanical aids, there are a number of most satisfactory ones on the market. One I like a lot is the "Relaxacizor" which gives you passive exercise. You don't do anything yourself—you let the "Relaxacizor" exercise your muscles. This will slim your waist and hips and firm your muscles but will not reduce your weight. The "Tiger Stretch" is again on the market. You have to work this yourself but it does fine things for your body if used regularly.

One of the best aids is the "Doorway Gym Bar," manufactured by the Olympian Industries in Chicago. This is for sale at Lewis and Conger in New York, and in sports shops throughout the country—it is a bar, with or without rings, to help you get limber and develop your muscles. I like it!

There are some mechanical massage machines—electrical and manual—that have some value, especially if you do not get professional massage.

If you have time and energy and enthusiasm, you may enjoy going to a gymnasium and getting a real work-out, complete with mechanical massage, hand massage, vapor baths and supervised exercise. If combined with your regulation high-protein diet—which I hope you're on this very minute—this will put you in fine condition in the shortest possible time. You won't get very far without your diet. Vapor baths take away moisture, so that, on the scales, you've lost several pounds. Drink four eight-ounce glasses of water or other liquids—you'll want them after the exercise and bath, too—and you'll drink the moisture right back again. But the exercise and massage—hand and mechanical—will firm you, and make you feel better, too. If your doctor thinks you are fit for it, and you want it, I would recommend, thoroughly, a course at a good gymnasium, complete with exercise and massage—you don't need to bother with the vapor baths. And please keep on your diet if you want to get results.

Probably you don't want such a strenuous work-out. The trip to a gymnasium, the dressing and undressing, and getting ready for the exercise wears me out just thinking about it. I couldn't take it. If you can, that's fine with me—if it is with you. In fact, hearty congratulations.

The exercise I recommend—the least amount of exercise you can have, and still do a thorough job of reduction—consists of fifteen minutes of bending and stretching every morning. You can do it at night, if you prefer—or if you miss it in the morning—but the morning is the best time. You'll feel fine afterwards. And fifteen minutes of exercise won't get you too hungry—you can eat your breakfast immediately afterwards and feel fine all day.

Why do you have to exercise? Because, being overweight and not exercising, you're undoubtedly flabby. And undoubtedly, too, you have a bad posture. Nearly all fat people are flabby and do not stand well. In fact, a lot of them are so fat that they've got themselves all out of shape—not only their outward layer of fat, which makes them look out of shape, but inner layers of fat around all of the organs of their bodies. More than that, they may actually have got their skeletons a bit awry—their backbones too curved, their ribs spread out. Their doctors may advise exercise and massage for special correction. If the whole body isn't badly distorted, simple exercises and diet will do the job.

Without exercise, and with diet only, as you get thin you'll get flabbier and flabbier. Your face will look drawn; as the fat disappears, the skin on your body may hang like a loose bag. Of course it may not be that bad at all. And with proper exercise—and not too much exercise, either—and with massage—even the massage you can give yourself, if you don't want to bother with a masseuse—you can get yourself in fine shape.

When you hear someone say, "Oh, she looks awful—

she's been dieting!" you can take it for granted that (a) the dieter did not have a good diet—she had one lacking in proteins and proper nutrients—and (b) she did not exercise as she lost weight. The people who get compliments are those who know what they're about, and do the right thing. After all, you've only got one body I Your body—your personal appearance—is all you have to present, outwardly, to the world. Why not be your best self? It's just as easy, once you put your mind to it. Determine to think yourself thin.

Exercise does not actually reduce you without dieting. All specialists, in either diet or exercise, will tell you that. But they will tell you that combining the two will produce remarkable results. Why not combine the two? Even fifteen minutes of proper exercise a day will tone your muscles. Turn them from being flabby to being properly firm. Firm muscles are the only ones that look well. You simply cannot have a good figure if your muscles are flabby, without tone, even if you are slender. Your stomach won't be flat and firm, you won't hold yourself properly or walk properly. Exercising will stimulate you, improve your metabolism. You can eat more of your proper diet, if your muscles are firm. Your skin will get over its flabby appearance, will firm, too.

But here is a warning: Do not exercise if you are very much overweight! Use mental discipline instead. Eat the right foods for you—and think yourself thin instead. Because, if you exercise while you are too fat, you may harden the fat and make it harder to lose. As you get nearer to normal, exercise will help a great deal. It will stimulate your system, help your metabolism and harden muscles. But get rid of the soft, flabby fat by diet first, while it is easier to lose. Then take a course of regular exercise, with or without accompaniment of mechanical exercisers.

They tell me that three S's are needed for slenderness. They are: Stretch, Shove and Shake. You stretch tall, you shove away from the table before you've had too much food, and you shake your head "No, no!" when offered a second helping. Very funny—as far as it goes. But, as usual with those seemingly bright epigrams, it doesn't go nearly far enough.

Certainly, the stretch part is good. You might start to stand and walk well, right this minute. Back up against a wall. With your backbone against it, that is, and your heels a few inches from the wall. Press the back of your head against the wall and as much of your backbone as you can. Now stretch tall! There I Then walk away from the wall. Keep that posture! Do that a dozen times a day, until standing straight is natural for you. Put a book on your head, if you like, and imagine you're in boarding school, getting a lesson in how to stand. Straighten out your knees when you walk, and put one foot in front of the other. Make tracks! Fat folks are inclined to keep their feet too far apart. They waddle. You won't, if you remember to stand straight and to put one foot in front of the other.

When walking, pretend you're a marionette, and that you're hanging from the ceiling by your ears. Stretch your neck and hold your head high. Walk that way I Before long, it will come natural to you.

One of the first signs of age is thrusting the head forward. Young folks hold their heads straight. Proud folks —beautiful people—hold their heads high and have lovely necklines. Shake your head from side to side, trying to push it backwards at each shake. Soon you'll have it in the right place. Keep it there.

Next, to use the good old army phrase, "Suck in your guts." Or, if you want to be a bit more elegant, use the phrase that all the little ladies use at the beauty parlors, "Tuck in your tummy." They both mean exactly the same thing. In other words, pretend that you're pressing your stomach against your backbone. Press it back! That will help firm your stomach muscle, help give you a good posture. *Stand straight! Stand high! Hold your head up as if it s on wires! Hold your stomach in!* You'll have to think to remember those. They are definitely part of the think yourself thin program, next to your mental attitude and your diet. If you get nothing more out of this book than learning how to stand and hold your head, you've got your money's worth! Folks have taken long courses in gymnasiums, and have come out with less. Holding yourself straight, your shoulders back, your head proud, your stomach in, will take years off your appearance. They will make you look pounds lighter! By practicing them until they become second nature— by thinking a good posture—you will have taken a fine step on the road ahead to a slender, young figure, a happy future.

You may want to use a tilted board, called variously "beauty boards," "beauty angles" and "glamour rests." These are boards raised, at one end, about 14 inches. Your head goes down, your feet up. You can buy these at dozens of shops—or you can have one made. Some folks use ironing boards. I think that's too narrow. Buying one is a good investment, if you use it. You can do several exercises on it—and it is good for you. There's no doubt of that! Get an angle board or any reclining chair on which you can lie with your head lower than your toes. Try to lie on it from twenty minutes to half an hour a day. You can relax. You can listen to the radio. You can even read, in a fashion. The blood runs to your head, and away from your feet. Your circulation is helped, and your face is given rejuvenation. It isn't magic—but it's a help.

You'll need other exercises for your face, too. Your face may look tired and not too young, already. When you diet and lose weight, it will probably look worse, unless you do something about it. Or you may have a round, young, smooth face before you diet, and look tired and older after you diet, as your face gets thinner—if you just forget it. You don't have to forget it.

First, wash your face every night and every morning with soap and water. Use any bland soap. I prefer a lanolin or cold cream soap, but any of the advertised soaps which you buy because you've been sold by the advertising will do. A very good soap is Baby Skin Oil Soap, which along with the Baby Skin Oil, is made by Mary Imogene Shepherd in Chicago. Both of these products are good. Lather your face well, using warm water. Then rinse all of the soap off, using only your hands. Rinse in very cold water. Then rub dry with a brisk, rough bath towel. Don't just pat with a smooth face towel. In fact, always use a bath towel for facial stimulation.

Next, apply an astringent. Both the washing and the astringent will give tone to the skin, help to overcome the looseness caused by the loss of fat. You can use any of the recognized astringents—or plain witch hazel. It's just as good! The others are quite all right—and highly priced. Plain witch hazel is good and not expensive. Any brand—I'm not backing any particular products now! But I've seen the laboratory analysis on dozens of beauty preparations and can guarantee that there are no secrets—nothing that will work wonders. The cheaper creams will do as well as the expensive ones, in everything but their psychological value. You read the advertisements—and you believe them. Or, in elegant surroundings, you're told by a clever saleswoman what the creams will do. If you can afford it, there's no reason why you shouldn't buy expensive creams, as long as you like them. Nivea Cream, an inexpensive product, is perfectly satisfactory. So are the plainer creams, made by houses such as Ponds or Hudnut or Coty. The expensive salon creams will serve you well too! The main thing is to keep your skin well oiled, after the astringent has dried. Every skin needs oil—especially the skin of persons who are losing weight. Use oil at night and in the morning, after you've washed your face with soap and water and rinsed it well.

Then, use a foundation, if you like, and a facial make-up. I'm sure I don't have to tell you how to make up your face!

Do your facial exercises night and morning, after you've applied the oil. Here are the best exercises, for the person who is dieting, to firm the muscles and help you look well, as the face loses fat.

1. Puff out your cheeks. Now, slap them smartly with your fingers, keeping the air in your cheeks. Do that for about one minute, after you're used to it. A few seconds, in the beginning.

2. Open your mouth as wide as you can. Keep your face tense. Now draw your mouth into a small O. Then stick your tongue out, holding your tongue in a point. If you look at yourself in the mirror, you won't seem at all pretty—but every muscle in your face will be exercised.

3. Pull your mouth to the left, then to the right. Then make circles with your lips, holding them closed. Hold the muscles tense.

4. With your thumbs and forefingers, start at the chin and go along the "edge" of your face—outline it by squeezing it in gentle little "takes," from the chin to below your ears. Pinch hard enough to bring the blood to the surface.

5. Press your lower lip up. Now chew, holding the muscles as taut as you can. You needn't let your jaws come quite together—your teeth shouldn't touch. Stretch your mouth as you chew. Try it with mouth open as well as closed. This will help face and neck muscles.

6. Same as 5, but press the inside of your hand, the thumb and lower palm, against your cheeks—and chew. Chew! Chew! You can harden the muscles of your face in this way, so that your cheeks will be smooth, even if you lose weight.

7. Put your two first fingers into your mouth. Press against the corners. Now, open and close your mouth, pulling hard with the fingers toward the corners. You won't stretch your mouth! On the contrary, you'll short en the muscles. Exercising is the only way to shorten muscles, you know.

8. Put your palms under your chin, with your fingers in front of your ears. Now chew, pushing your palms upwards, against your chin, but holding the rest of your hands against your face.

9. Hold your lips together. Press hard. Now press your lips upwards and screw up your face. Hold the muscles tense.

10. Purse your lips into a pout. Open your eyes and lift your eyebrows. Tense the muscles.

11. Turn your head from side to side, muscles tense.

12. Turn your head in a complete circle, muscles tense.

There you are! The Big Dozen facial exercises. Undoubtedly you've read of others. You can add those to your program.

A little massage won't hurt your face. Too much of it may stretch the skin. Massage upwards with the fingers. Then wipe the oil off your face. In the morning, after your bath, you'll be ready for make-up. Last thing at night, add just a little more cream—not enough to look ugly or to soil the bed clothes—and you're ready for bed.

Try to sleep without a pillow. The harder the bed, the better for you. Have your room well ventilated, but have a lot of covers, or an electric blanket, so your body is comfortable and warm. How many hours do you sleep? If you're trying to reduce, you probably can cut down on your sleep. I used to sleep eight hours. Now I sleep five or six. And I feel a lot better—and look better, too. And think of those extra hours I have for reading or working or having fun! I'm writing this at two o'clock in the morning—a fine time for working. No telephone calls! No interruptions! No place to go! Just grand for relaxation or reading—or working. Earlier in the evening, I can go out and have fun.

You'll want body exercises, too. Again, I can't invent any new magic ones that will reduce you overnight. Wish I could! One good exercise I like is to stretch your head, as high as you can stretch. Head up. Stretch and stretch!

I know other exercises, too. And I wanted the best for you. So I went to the source. To Monte MacLevy. You know about MacLevy. He's the head of about 130 reduction gymnasiums—slenderizing salons. For forty years, he's been reducing people. He figures he's taken over eight million pounds from two million people. Quite a lot of reducing! Thirty-two of the salons are in New York. The others are all over the world, under the MacLevy name. He also runs a health farm, and he now has dancing schools for children, too. He took time out of his busy day, with about half of his 2,600 employees clamoring to see him, and in the midst of planning television shows, to give me exercises for you.

He gave me six exercises. Says they'll do the job—condition you, make your muscles firm. If you diet and then exercise for fifteen minutes a day, he says, you'll be surprised at the results. Not in a day or two, perhaps. But try the exercises for a month. Then you'll want to go on.

You should have stood in bed! Well, you can't stand in bed, with these exercises. But you can lie in bed! You'll feel a lot better than if you had to jump up immediately. Three of these exercises—the first three—can be done in bed, or on the floor. The other three are standing exercises.

After your exercises, you might want a massage. You can massage yourself. Around your waist and in the back, where you are fat, you can learn to "wring yourself out." Grab hold of yourself—take a fold of your flesh, as if it were a thick piece of rope. Then work this flesh as if you could squeeze the fat out of it. Then go on to the rest of your body—wherever the fat is loose enough to grasp. Slap the flesh firmly, too, until you're pink from the slaps. Perhaps not as good as a professional massage! I get the same results. The Oster Massage Instrument is fine as a "self-help" electric massage machine.

Then you'll be ready for your hot and cold bath and rub down. Ready to start the day in the right way. You'll feel fine.

Don't forget to weigh yourself—and mark down your

weight. Don't forget, at night, to write down what you've eaten during the day, and check up the calories and proteins to see that you have eaten the right foods, and haven't exceeded your diet. Then, forget all about the diet and the exercise—except at meal time, or when it is necessary for you to think about meals. Turn your thoughts to other things—to some of the interesting things you'll find, once you've put your mind to it. Even your work will seem more interesting, if you're feeling fit, and have become alert and eager to learn about everything you can.

Mr. MacLevy has written a very good book, containing dozens of exercises. It is called *Pounds* O|f, and you may want to purchase it, if you want more exercises than I can give you here. Those I give you will do the job—they're all that are necessary for thinking yourself thin. But you may be ambitious and want more. Two other books with very fine exercises that I can recommend are *New Bodies For Old* by Dorothy Nye, published by Funk & Wagnalls, and *Body Control,* by Herman Gawer, M.A., Supervisor of Health Guidance, City College of New York, and Herbert Michaelman, with a Foreword by Dr. Harold M. Erickson, State Health Officer of Oregon.

Here, then, are your MacLevy exercises, chosen especially for you, for as rapid as possible firming and reduction, to be used while you're thinking—and dieting—yourself thin. Start off doing each exercise twice. Increase until you're doing each one 25 times. Then bend and stretch for the rest of your fifteen minutes.

EXERCISE I

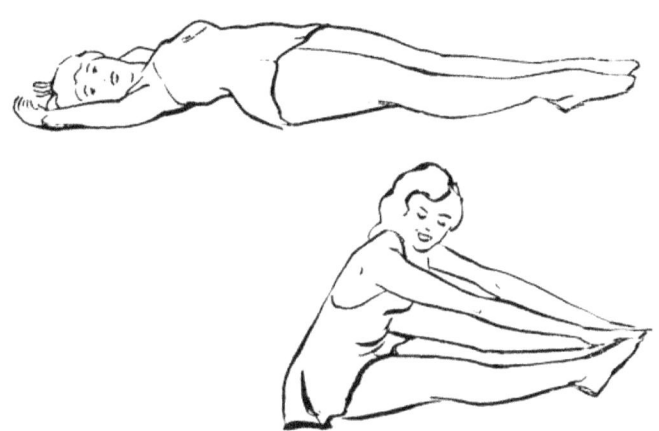

AT THE START ....Lie on the back, legs together, arms stretched out over head.

COUNT one.....................Swing forward to a sitting position, letting the arms lead. Bend forward until the hands touch the toes.

      two ....Return to the starting position, back leading, arms following straight overhead.

REPEAT ....Five times. *Very slow.*

BENEFITS ....This limbering exercise produces quick results in conditioning upper back and spine, and in reducing stomach.

SPECIAL
  INSTRUCTIONS.........If it is difficult to come up from the floor, brace the feet under a couch or heavy chair. Avoid bending knees.

EXERCISE 2

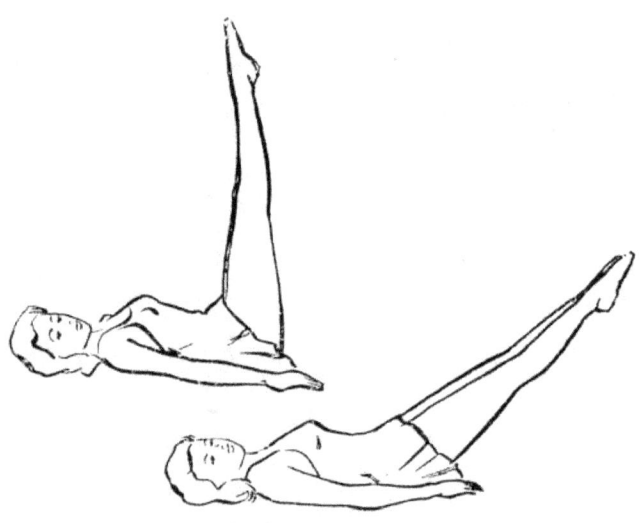

AT THE START ....Lie on the back, legs together, arms at the sides.

COUNT one .... Raise both legs straight into the air, keeping toes pointed and knees straight.

two ....Lower legs slowly to the floor.

REPEAT ....Five times. *Slow.*

BENEFITS ....This exercise is good for the thighs, but the concentrated exercise is on the stomach muscles.

SPECIAL
INSTRUCTIONS __ When lowering the legs, take care not to let them drop with a thud the last half of the way. Keep toes pointed. Avoid bending knees and hooking feet.

EXERCISE 3

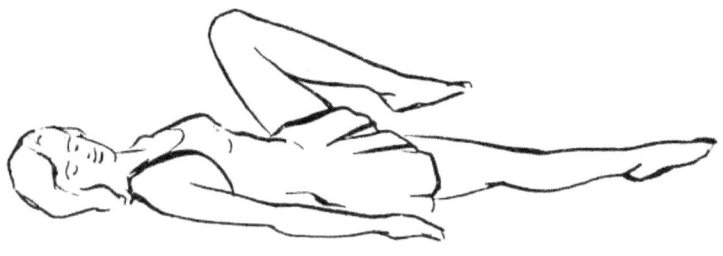

AT THE START............ Lie on the back, knees to chest, arms at the sides.

COUNT one.................... Thrust the right leg forward, knee straight, within two inches of the floor.

two.................... Bring the right knee back to the chest quickly.

three .... Repeat with the left leg.

four .... Return to starting position.

REPEAT.......................... Ten times. *Rapid.*

BENEFITS...................... The stomach gets major help from this exercise, although legs and rear are also benefited.

SPECIAL
INSTRUCTIONS........ Keep the knees straight when the legs are extended, and do not let the heels touch the floor. Avoid doing this exercise too slowly.

EXERCISE 4

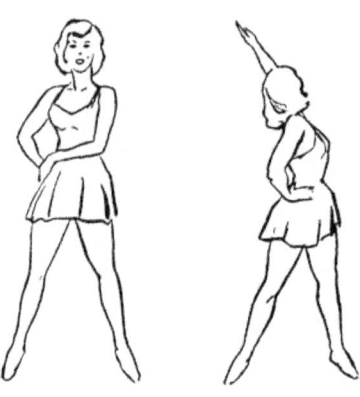

AT THE START............ Stand astride, right hand on hip, left hand on top of right hand.

COUNT one.................... Fling left hand sideward over head, twisting torso as far to left as possible.

two.................... Return left hand to starting position on top of right.

REPEAT...........................Ten times and reverse, using right arm. *Slow.*

BENEFITS...................... This exercise conditions shoulders, arms, and bust, and starts the work of reducing waist. It is fine for the spine.

SPECIAL
INSTRUCTIONS .... When the hand goes up, stretch backward as far as possible; the head will turn naturally with the shoulders. Let the head turn as far as possible, but keep it level, chin up. Be sure to get the arm well up over the head. Avoid bending the elbow.

EXERCISE 5

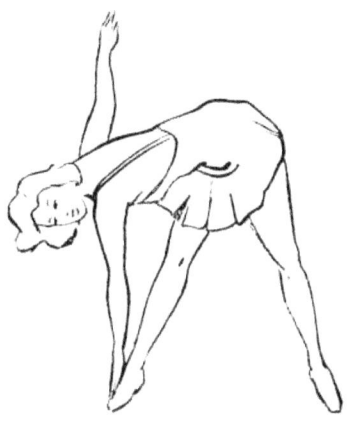

AT THE START ....Stand erect, feet astride, arms out stretched to side, shoulder level.

COUNT one ....Twist trunk to the right and touch the left hand to the right toe.

    two....................Return to starting position.

    three ....Twist trunk to the left, and touch the right hand to the left toe.

    four...................Return to starting position.

REPEAT ....Ten times.

BENEFITS ....This limbers the waist, aids the reducing of shoulders and arms, and tightens the abdominal muscles.

SPECIAL
INSTRUCTIONS.........Keep an easy rhythm. All bending exercises should be easy, not jerky. Keep the knees straight. Avoid letting the shoulders slump forward.

Exercise 6

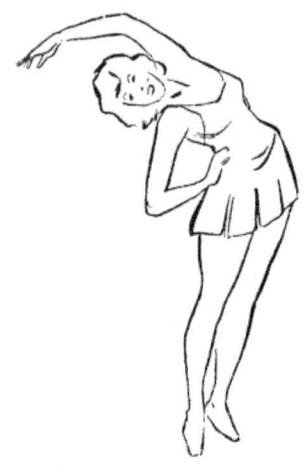

AT THE START .... Stand erect, feet astride, right arm on right hip, left arm completely relaxed over the head.

COUNT one to four .... Bend torso as far as possible to the right and, using a bouncing motion on each count, stretch farther and farther down for four counts.

      five to eight ... Make a quick reverse between counts, and do the same exercise to the left.

REPEAT .... Five times. *Rapid.*

BENEFITS .... Especially good for reducing hips and waist.

SPECIAL
   INSTRUCTIONS   ___Keep the arm which is hooked over the head completely relaxed. Let head relax during bouncing motions. Avoid tensing the neck muscles.

CHAPTER 24

Sweets
to the sweet

ONE OF THE MOST pleasant things about reducing is talking with other people on diets, and exchanging recipes. From experts to amateurs, everyone who is losing weight has a pet diet or a pet recipe to talk about. Some of the ideas are grand! Some of them. . . .Well, I said some were grand!

That's why I don't like to compare overweights with alcoholics. Overweights love to talk about food—and the food they can eat. Alcoholics, if they're on the wagon, like to talk about the fact that they can't drink at all. In fact, their fight is against all drinking. Folks who weigh too much do not, actually, have much of a problem. They don't have to give up the pleasures of the table. They just have to learn which pleasures they can accept with pleasure.

All food is fattening! The idea is to chose food that is the least fattening and the most helpful. Which usually means food very low in calories and, if possible, high in proteins. Sometimes, food has both qualities—and is perfect. Sometimes it's one or the other—and that's fair enough.

The trouble with most low-calorie foods is that they aren't low caloried enough. In choosing low-calorie foods —and recipes for low-calorie food—the idea is to chose those that are the lowest—and still delicious. And that's not too easy. In fact, recently, in one of New York's best newspapers, a staff writer gave recipes with the heading "Low in Cost, Low in Calories," and one of the items given was a dessert which was 234 calories per portion, minus topping, and consisted mostly of dried prunes —a very high-calorie fruit. Another dessert contained 185 calories per portion. That's not what I call low-calorie foods! So don't just choose a dish because it's called low-calorie. Study it for yourself. You've got your table! A main dish, high in proteins, may cost you as many as 350 calories of the 1,000 or 1,200 calories that you have to spend for the day. No luncheon dish should cost you more than 200 of your calories; no auxiliary dish more than 100 calories. In fact, outside of your main high-calorie dish, 100 for the accompanying dish is a good average—and a lot of dishes should be much lower.

This chapter isn't a full and rounded cook book. I wish it were! Maybe, some day, I'll gather enough good, low-calorie recipes to publish a whole book of them. I'd like that. But for the present, I'll contribute a few I've worked out myself, or friends have given me. They'll give you ideas—start you on your own experiments, your own hunt for good recipes.

As a matter of fact, you don't need a lot of recipes to be on a successful high-protein, low-calorie diet. The diet is too   simple to need many recipes—and it may still be varied. Meats can be cooked simply. Vegetables should be cooked simply. High-protein breads can be purchased better than they can be baked at home. Desserts can be made without much trouble. Too many other dishes are unnecessary. You'll get all of the recipes you'll need to begin a successful diet regime and think yourself thin with no trouble at all.

First, I'll give you the names of some cook books that may help you. I collect cook books—I love 'em!—and these are about the best I have with low-calorie recipes in them. But even these have to be looked over carefully. There isn't one of them that doesn't have recipes that I consider much too high in calories for the person on a careful, thoughtful diet. That's where you must use your own judgment. I'm taking it for granted that now you know enough about foods—and about your own needs—so you can use discrimination in choosing things for yourself, for your family and for your guests.

The Reducing Cook Book and Diet Guide, by Llewellyn Miller, with a foreword by Dr. Morris Fishbein, and published by Fawcett, is an excellent book that you'll want, I'm sure. It contains 500 recipes for the overweight person.

Paul Bragg's Health Cook Book, by Paul C. Bragg, published by Alfred Knopf, is full of fine recipes—all good for you, though it is not a reduction cook book. Some of them are good for you now. Some of them are good for you after you've reached your normal weight, and can add a few hundred more calories to your meals.

Reducer's Cook Book, by Ann Williams-Heller, published by Wilfred Funk, is a fine beginner's book, for it teaches you a great many things about buying, about planning and about serving diet meals. It gives good menus, too. Like most cook books of this type, it is "padded" in order to make a full book—a lot of the recipes are too simple, or are not particularly low in calories—but the book is written with taste and understanding, and the dieter can profit by it.

The Hamburger Cook Book, by Esther K. Schwartz and Ruth Kooperman, published by Abelard Press, is most useful, as hamburger is high in protein—and the recipes are well planned.

Diabetic Menus, Meals And Recipes, by Betty M. West, published by Doubleday, is just what the title says it is. So many of the recipes are not for the dieter, because they contain too much fat—which is allowed for the diabetic. However, a great many of them are suitable. Saccharin is used instead of sugar, and the values of each dish are given—carbohydrates, fats and the entire protein contents—so it is excellent, too, for the inexperienced cook. You know just what you're getting in every recipe.

The Salt-Free Diet Cook Book, by Dr. Emil G. Conason and Ella Metz, will be valuable if you're cutting down your salt intake, because the dishes are full of flavor and the recipes are carefully worked out, with their sodium and caloric values given.

The Gayelord Hauser Cook Book, published by Coward McCann, is not as scientifically planned as the above books, but some of the recipes are low in calories and many of them are delicious—fine recipes for the discriminating diner—and full of good ideas on the preparing of food, especially vegetables, organ meats and meat substitutes. It is not specifically for reduction, so you must use your own judgment.

201 Tasty Dishes For Reducers, with the Victor Lindlahr seven-day reducing diet, published by the Journal of Living, at the Country Life Press, contains recipes that will add variety to your diet—if you're looking for variety.

The Salad Book, by Louis P. De Gouy, published by Greenberg, is not a diet book at all, but because salads are good for dieters, this book contains many excellent recipes that can be used—if you pick them with care.

Let's Cook It Right, by Adelle Davis, published by Harcourt Brace, is again definitely not a diet book, but a book with fine and wholesome recipes, from which you can choose any number that are suitable for low-calorie, high-protein diets.

Two slim books, both published in England but for sale here, may add variety to your meals. One is *Food For Health,* by Jessie R. Thomson, of the Edinburgh School of Natural Therapeutics, and published by Thomson Publishers; the other, *Fruit Dishes And Raw Vegetables,* by Drs. M. Bircher-Benner and Max E. Bircher, giving the well-known Bircher-Benner method of preparing and serving fruits and vegetables.

The South American Gentleman's Companion, in two volumes, one devoted to exotic cookery and the other to exotic drinks, by Charles H. Baker, Jr., and published by

Crown, contains a number of recipes that are unusual, and low in calories, and drinks that contain no alcohol, too, together with a novel diet that adds cider vinegar to the daily menus.

Your own favorite cook book will contain a lot of recipes you can use—if you'll hunt for them, discarding all that are high in carbohydrates and fats. A difficult task, but fun, too. And think how pleased you'll be when you make your own discoveries!

In giving you my recipes, I shall make no attempt to classify them, or even to give their correct caloric value. You can work that out for yourself, if you're interested. You'll be able to see, from the ingredients, just what they contain, and why they're good for you. They're all low in calories, and usually high in proteins.

First, then, my Magicream, because I think you'll like it. And because you may want to try it right away, and not leaf through the pages, looking for it. It's very simple, and it can help solve your dessert problem, the most difficult problem of the dieter. It can also be used as a salad dressing. As a dessert, the caloric value will run from 50 to 100 calories per portion, depending on what you add to it and the size of your portions. You must follow the recipe exactly if you want it to be 3 success. My present to you!

I. THINK YOURSELF THIN MAGICREAM

2   cups of skimmed milk. *This must be fat-free.*

2   envelopes unsweetened gelatin.

That's all, for the basic recipe! You see it contains

twice as much gelatin as you usually use for that amount of liquid. Good for you, too—high in protein and minerals.

Into the cold milk put the contents of both envelopes of gelatin. Do not dissolve them first I Just dump them in! With a rotary beater, beat until foamy. Put on the stove, over a very low heat, and beat constantly until the mixture is luke warm—warm enough to dissolve the gelatin. It will thicken as you beat it. When it is just warm, take it off the stove and continue to beat until it is the consistency of thick whipped cream. That's all I

If you wish to use this as a dessert, add saccharin or Sucaryl tablets while it is on the stove, so they will dissolve. I use 10 tablets for 2 cups of milk. Add a bit of your salt substitute and a teaspoon of vanilla.

This tastes like a whipped cream dessert, to which white of egg has been added. I serve it to my guests. They don't know what is in it—and they like it.

If you like, you may add fresh fruits to the Magicream and put it into the refrigerator. Or you may serve it at once. It will thicken a bit in the refrigerator, and may be put into molds. Strawberries are especially good in it. Peaches are good, too. If your diet is progressing favorably and you want to treat yourself, you may add split ladyfingers. Put them around the inside of a glass and add the Magicream. You'll have a very nice Charlotte Russe. The plain cream, flavored with Sucaryl and vanilla, makes an excellent dessert—one you won't tire of quickly, and a welcome change from fruit or cheese—

usually the only "allowed" desserts. This may be frozen in your ice tray for an odd, spongy and very good dessert. If you wish to use it as a salad dressing, add a bit of Sucaryl—one tablet—a teaspoon of mustard, and the juice of one or two lemons. It is excellent with fish, cucumbers or aspic.

2. THINK YOURSELF THIN SOUR CREAM OR CREAM CHEESE

This is my second-best recipe. I'm sure, if you're a gourmet, you like sour cream and butter—two delicacies forbidden on your diet. This near-sour cream will substitute for both of them. I invented it, too. You may also use it as cream cheese. And I eat it every day. So do my guests. In fact, I seldom serve butter at all, and I never buy sour cream any more—a saving in money and calories. This is simple, too.

I pound of pot cheese.

¾ cup of buttermilk.

And that's all! Put the pot cheese—which is the lowest cheese in caloric value that you can buy, or cottage cheese, if you can't buy pot cheese, together with the buttermilk in your Waring Blender or electric mixer, and mix well. Use a hand beater, if you haven't one of the others. That's all! You'll get a thick, creamy mixture that tastes so much like sour cream it takes an expert to tell the difference. The difference is all in the calories! This will make a thick mixture, which can be spread on your high-protein bread or crackers, as if it were cream cheese or butter. If you want to make it thinner, to use over fruit or salad, add more buttermilk. It will keep for a week in the refrigerator. Maybe it will last longer than that. Mine is always eaten up long before then.

3. THINK YOURSELF THIN CHEESE SPREAD When I wrote about "cheese spread substitutes" in the menus, this is what I meant. When you dine out and want cheese, you'll have to eat the real thing. But dining at home, you can eat this substitute, which is much lower in calories, but good in proteins. It is made like the sour cream mixture.

1 pound pot cheese.
1 cup of buttermilk (a little less if it doesn't get too thick to mix).
1/3 pound Roquefort cheese—or your favorite cheese. 1 small onion.
1 clove of garlic.
1 envelope gelatin.
1 scant tablespoon Worcestershire Sauce.
Salt substitute.

Mince onion and garlic—the powdered may be used if you would rather use them. Add the other ingredients, with gelatin heated in part of milk. Beat in mixer or by hand. That's all! This makes a delicious cheese spread, which grows better after a couple of days in the refrigerator, when the stronger cheese has a chance to blend. If you have a difficult time mixing it, leave it in a warm room until the cheese becomes softer and easier to handle. You may use cheddar, if you prefer the flavor. A bit of this cheese, with an apple, makes a fine "extra meal" dish, or a dessert. It can be used to stuff celery or small tomatoes, too.

One of my favorite dishes—for breakfast, as a snack in the afternoon, as a dessert, or before I go to bed at night—is cream cheese, preserves, and buttered toast. I can't have that. But I can have a very good substitute— so good, in fact, that I don't miss the original at all. For toast, I use a slice of artichoke or gluten bread or toast. For the cream cheese, I use the spread made from pot cheese and buttermilk I've just told you about in recipe No. 2. And here is the recipe for preserves. It is the best I've found for a low-calorie sweet of this type.

4. THINK YOURSELF THIN PRESERVES

1 pint—two cupfuls—of fruit, sliced.
¾ cup water.
14 Sucaryl tablets.
2 saccharin tablets.
1 envelope gelatin or 2 tablespoons powdered pectin.

You can use any fruit for this. Strawberries are best, and even in winter you can treat yourself to a pint of strawberries. If you use apples, add a bit of nutmeg and cinnamon for flavoring. If you want to make old-fashioned apple butter, substitute cider or apple juice for water. Plums and pears make good preserves, too. If you want to make orange marmalade, use thin-skinned oranges, soak in water for a while, and then add fresh water before cooking. Grape juice may also be used.

Boil the fruit with ½ cup of water for five minutes. Add the Sucaryl tablets and the gelatin or pectin, which has been dissolved in ¼, cup cold water. Boil rapidly for two minutes. Take oft stove, and, when slightly cooled, add saccharin for an additional "step-up" sweetener. This makes two glasses. A portion of this, with the No. 2 diet cream cheese and toast, is about 50 calories— a good, low-calorie sweet dessert.

5. YOGURT

Here is the simplest way I know to make yogurt. This is low-calorie yogurt. Yogurt won't do any magic things for you, but it's good for you. So is buttermilk!

Put into a bowl:

1 quart of skimmed milk.
¼ cup regular bought whole-milk yogurt.

Heat until cooking thermometer registers 120^0 F., or is just good and warm, when you test it. Cover and keep warm—90^0 to 110° F. If you have a pilot light on your gas stove, put the bowl over the pilot light, and cover with regular cover and then bath towel. It will be thick in about three hours. Test it. When thick enough, put in refrigerator. You can use some of this to start the next batch, starting with new culture every few weeks. If you like a thicker yogurt, add ½ cup of powdered skimmed milk.

6. FRUIT JUICE SPONGE

You may call this what you like. A friend of mine

calls it Bavarian Cream—and guests think it is made with cream and eggs. It's low in calories, delicious as a dessert. Serve it plain, or add fresh or canned fruit. Fruit salad, canned without sugar—the water- or juice-packed variety—is especially good with this.

1 No. 2 can of pineapple juice—my preference—
or 2 cupfuls of any fresh fruit juice.
8 Sucaryl or saccharin tablets.
2 envelopes gelatin.
⅓ cup cottage or pot cheese.

You may add a bit of salt or salt substitute, or a bit of nutmeg, if you like. Add the gelatin to the juice. Beat with rotary beater. Heat until the gelatin is dissolved. Beat again. Add the sweetener—which may be more or less, according to your taste. Then add cottage or pot cheese and beat until the cheese has dissolved. This will be a pale, opaque cream. Put into refrigerator, and when slightly thickened, add the fruit—if you want fruit. It isn't necessary, for it's a very nice dessert as is. Use one envelope of gelatin, beat and freeze for a good sherbet, a fine summer dessert. You may add the beaten white of an egg for a smoother sherbet.

7. BAKED APPLES

Here is an old favorite that may be adapted to diets. Choose any good apples. Hollow out the centers. Fill centers with a mixture of gluten bread crumbs, chopped apple, a few raisins, a chopped nut or two—or you may omit this—cinnamon and nutmeg. Over this pour ¼ cup of water, in which Sucaryl or saccharin tablets have been dissolved, for every four apples. Put in pan in which there's enough water to keep the apples from sticking. Bake about half an hour, or until tender. These are good hot or cold. You may add a little "sour cream mixture," recipe No. 2, on top, for a special dessert.

8. APPLE PIE

Here is a very good apple pie substitute. If it doesn't taste too much like apple pie, I'm sure you won't mind— for it is good, and very low in calories. You'll need:

Apples.
Gelatin.
Sucaryl or saccharin to taste.
Cottage cheese or "cream cheese substitute," No. 2.
Low-calorie crumbs.
A bit of salt substitute, nutmeg and cinnamon, if
    you like them in pies.

Mash the crumbs with a rolling pin or smooth drinking glass. Spread evenly in a pie pan. Cook sliced and peeled apples in ½ cup of water until just tender. Add sweetener and envelope of gelatin, which has been dissolved in a little water. Add seasoning. Now there are two things you may do. You may pour this directly on the crumbs and add a topping of cream mixture No. 1, or No. 2. Or you may put the cream directly into the mixture and mix it well. The flavors- will be quite different, giving you two varieties. Or you may leave the apple mixture plain, for an open-faced plain apple pie.

Put in the refrigerator until cool and firm. The mixture alone, without the crumbs, will make a good, non-fattening apple sauce.

A plain apple sauce can, of course, be made with just the apples, water and sweetener. But you'll like the apple pie, I'm sure. It will add variety to your diet.

9. CHEESE PIE

Here is another dessert you'll like for a change, I'm sure. Not as low in calories as the other desserts—and cheese pie isn't one of my favorite desserts, anyhow. But if it's one of yours, there's no reason why you won't enjoy this.

½ cup low-calorie crumbs.
2 eggs, separated.
15 Sucaryl tablets.
2 cups cottage or pot cheese.
1 teaspoon lemon juice.
½ teaspoon grated lemon rind.
¼ cup skimmed milk or buttermilk.
A bit of cinnamon.

Spread crumbs on bottom of oiled and floured pie pan. Dissolve Sucaryl in milk. Add to cottage cheese and flavorings. Beat yolk of eggs and add. Beat again. Then add beaten egg white and fold in. Bake at 350° F. for about 35 minutes. This has been praised as a good low-calorie dessert.

10. CHOCOLATE WHIPPED CREAM PIE

This has no chocolate in it, and no whipped cream

either, so perhaps the title isn't quite exact. But it's a fairly low-calorie dessert, and may be served occasionally.

> ½ cup low-calorie crumbs.
> 2 ounces low-calorie cocoa—buy at health store.
> 1 envelope plain gelatin.
> ¼ cup cold water.
> 1 cup skimmed milk.
> 2 eggs, separated.
> 15 Sucaryl tablets.
> 1 teaspoon vanilla.
> Imitation whipped cream, No. 1 or No. 2.

This dessert may be served as a custard, instead of a pie. I like it better in pie form.

Spread crumbs on bottom of pie pan. They won't be much like a pie crust, but they will add body to the dessert.

Put the gelatin in cold water until dissolved. Scald milk in double boiler. Add cocoa. Beat until smooth. Add Sucaryl and beat again. Add well-beaten egg yolks and cook until mixture thickens—about five minutes. Add gelatin and vanilla. Take from fire, and, when slightly cool, fold in well-beaten egg white. Put into refrigerator. Before serving, spread with one of your two special creams—the Magicream, or the sour cream mixture, whichever you prefer. Or use a mixture of pot cheese, gelatin and plain milk, instead of buttermilk, which is good, too.

II. CHIFFON PIE

The reason I'm going in so heavily for desserts is that they are the most neglected items on the menus of overweights. "Limit your desserts to fresh fruits," you're told, because the advisor doesn't know anything else. You can find other desserts, too, if you'll hunt for them. Chiffon pies—almost like the real ones—can be made with low caloric value, though not quite as low as some of the other desserts I've told you about.

I'll give the rules for lemon chiffon pie, but you may want to use strawberries or pineapple—canned, if you prefer.

> 1 envelope plain gelatin.
> 1/4 cup cold water.
> 1/3 cup lemon juice
> 3 eggs, separated.
> ½ teaspoon lemon rind.
> 15 Sucaryl tablets,

Dissolve gelatin in cold water. In top of boiler put beaten egg yolks, lemon juice, a bit of salt or salt substitute, Sucaryl and gelatin. Cook until of custard consistency. Add grated lemon peel. Cool, and added beaten egg white. Pour onto crumbs and chill.

12. EGGLESS CHIFFON PIE

You can make an eggless chiffon pie, too. Here it is, in coffee flavor:

Dissolve 15 tablets of Sucaryl and 2 teaspoons of instant coffee in ¾ cup of boiling water. Add 1 tablespoon of flour. Cook until mixture is well dissolved. Cool and add ¼ teaspoon of vanilla. Add 1 envelope gelatin, dissolved in ½ cup of water, and beat until fluffy. Add ½ portion Magicream No. 1. Chill. Before serving, spread top with the other half of Magicream recipe.

13. DRY SKIMMED MILK POWDER WHIPPED CREAM

You may use this as a whipped cream topping, instead of the Magicream, if you prefer. You'll need:

> 1 tablespoon lemon juice.
> ½ teaspoonful vanilla.
> ½ cup dry skimmed milk powder.
> 6 tablets Sucaryl or saccharin.

Put ½ cup of water into mixing bowl. Add lemon juice, sweetening tablets and vanilla. Sprinkle on the milk powder. Beat until stiff—preferably with electric beater. This will take about ten minutes. Put in refrigerator for half an hour before using. This can be used in any recipe that calls for whipped cream.

Fruit gelatins are the standby of the dieters. Because they are more common, I haven't given them until now. Made with unsweetened gelatin, they are good—and good for you. You may add whole fruit and have a fancier dessert. By using "whipped cream" topping No. 1, N0.2 or No. 13, they become festive enough for company or special occasions. Here are some of the best. You can work out others, yourself.

14. LEMON GELATIN

Grated rind of one lemon.

1½ cups boiling water.

1 envelope gelatin.

¼ cup cold water.

4 tablespoons lemon juice.

12 tablets saccharin or Sucaryl.

Boil lemon rind and water for two minutes. Soften gelatin in cold water. Add to hot liquid and stir until dissolved. Add lemon juice and saccharin. Strain into molds and chill until set. Add fruits for variety.

15. GRAPE JUICE GELATIN

1 envelope gelatin.

¼ cup cold water.

1 cup hot water.

½ cup grape juice.

1 tablespoon lemon juice.

1½ tablets saccharin or Sucaryl.

Soften gelatin in cold water. Add hot water and stir until dissolved. Add grape juice, lemon juice and saccharin. Pour into molds and chill. To serve, dip the mold in hot water, then turn out on serving dish. Or—when gelatin mixture is nearly set, beat until frothy, then pour into molds.

16. GRAPE SPONGE

Make up recipe for grape juice gelatin.

2 egg whites.

When gelatin is nearly set, beat until frothy. Beat egg whites until stiff and fold into gelatin. Pour into molds and chill.

17. FRUIT GELATIN

    1 envelope gelatin.
  ¼ cup cold water.
  1½ cups boiling water.
  ¼ cup lemon juice.
    Grated rind of one lemon.
    12 tablets saccharin or Sucaryl.
    6 sections orange.
    6 sections grapefruit.

Boil water and rind for two minutes. Soften gelatin in cold water. Add to hot lemon liquid and stir until dissolved. Add lemon juice and saccharin, stir, strain and chill. Cut each section of fruit into three pieces. When jelly is nearly set, stir in cut fruit, mold, chill until firm and serve plain, or with one of the cream substitutes. Strawberries may be substituted for citrus fruit.

18. SPANISH CREAM

    1 envelope gelatin.

  ¼ cup cold water.
    1 cup milk.
  ¾ cup boiling water.
    2 eggs, separated.
  1½ teaspoons vanilla.
  ¼ teaspoon salt.
    6 tablets saccharin or Sucaryl.

Heat water and milk over boiling water. Soften gelatin in cold water. Add to hot milk mixture and stir until lemon colored. Stir gelatin mixture slowly into egg yolks. Return to stove and cook over boiling water until mixture begins to thicken. Remove from stove, add vanilla and salt and chill. Beat egg whites until stiff and fold into jelly when almost set. Mold and chill until firm.

19. BUTTERMILK CUSTARD

½ cup water.
2 cups buttermilk.
1 envelope gelatin.
Saccharin or Sucaryl to taste. I use 10 tablets.

Dissolve gelatin in water. Add buttermilk. Heat until gelatin is dissolved. Add sweetening. Beat in electric beater. Put on ice. Delicious—and you'd never guess how it was made. Fine alone or with stewed fruit.

So you see, there are a lot of good desserts that can be served on low-calorie diets. You'll find others, too, I'm sure.

There's one candy I can tell you about. Marshmallows. Perhaps not as good as the big, luscious, plump ones you can buy in any confectionery shop—but most satisfactory if you aren't eating regulation sweets.

20. DIET MARSHMALLOWS

4 envelopes of gelatin.
2 cups of skimmed milk, absolutely non-fat.
12 Sucaryl or saccharin tablets.
Vanilla.
A bit of salt or salt substitute.

Stir the gelatin into the milk. Beat hard. Add sweetening tablets, salt, vanilla. Heat over a low flame, while beating the cream every minute. Beat until stiff. When stiff, and sweetener and gelatin are thoroughly dissolved, pour into a floured pan. Put into refrigerator. Cut into inch-sized squares, roll in flour, and serve. A low-caloried candy I think you'll enjoy. You may flavor it with peppermint or cocoa, too, or roll it in cocoa.

Now you have a good start on sweets, usually the one item that is missing from the dieter's menus. These, with plain fruit or cheese, will give you a variety of good things to eat as your last course at dinner, when you dine at home, with the marshmallows and cream spreads for "nibbles"

CHAPTER 25

Keep on eating

MEAT IS THE CHIEF ITEM on the menus of most folks on reduction diets. And most of the ways of cooking meats are quite satisfactory for the dieters. You can't, of course, eat breaded meats or meats that have added sauces. But plain meats, well cooked, are fine for you. Follow your favorite cook book.

21. THINK YOURSELF THIN DRY FRY Fried meats are the easiest and quickest to prepare. Unfortunately, they've fallen into disgrace. Hard to digest. Takes too much fat to make them palatable. However, if you use the "dry fry" method, I think you'll find that frying will not add a great deal of fat to your food, and that the food will be palatable and digestible.

The dry fry method is my own idea, as far as I can find out. So it's a real Think Yourself Thin method of cooking.

The first part isn't my own invention at all! Get a package of "Pantastic," a patent preparation made by Processed Surfaces, Inc., in Memphis and New York.

This is for sale in hardware and department stores—you can coat your frying pans with this, so that you do not have to use much fat for cooking. One application stays on for a couple of weeks—and a new application can then be applied. The directions are on the package. Use it only for your frying pans, so it will last a long time.

Now, take a lump of butter about the size of a walnut. Unsalted butter is preferred, if you're on a low-salt diet. Make this lump into a round ball and put it on ice until it's firm. Take a clean cloth—an old handkerchief or bit of cheesecloth will do. Make a swab, putting the butter in the center of the cloth, and twisting it around. Keep on ice. When you're ready to fry, heat the pan, and rub the swab over the surface of the pan. That's all! You may use a paint brush, if you use a liquid vegetable oil for frying instead of butter. Small steaks, chops, eggs, hamburgers—almost anything can be fried by this dry fry method.

Another method of frying without too much fat is to use a piece of bacon, and rub the pan with this. This is good when frying kidneys or liver. Or put a little water in your frying pan.

If your doctor allows you to use mineral oil, it is quite satisfactory for frying. If you wish it to have a good flavor, add a few tablespoons of olive oil, or your favorite vegetable oil, to each pint of mineral oil. Then you can use it for salads or for frying.

After you have fried the food the way you want it, take it out of the pan, and add a little water, some Worcestershire Sauce or Savita or Boveril, and make a good gravy.

If meat and potatoes are your favorite foods, boil one potato, slicing it before boiling. When the potato is tender, put it into the gravy, and cook until the gravy has been absorbed. Add Accent, and a sprinkling of parsley and salt substitute.

22. ROAST MEATS

I don't have to tell you how to prepare those! Use your favorite recipe. If you can afford them, you'll ask for nothing better than roast meats. I think you'll find the most satisfactory way will be to roast the meat in an uncovered pan, meat side up. Add black pepper, a very little salt, garlic and onions. Do not add flour or extra fat.

You may not be able to afford roast beef, or any of the other regulation roasts, too often. I know I can't. The standby could be one of the less expensive cuts, in pot roasts, short ribs, or stews. Beef heart is most satisfactory, too, if properly prepared. So is tongue, fresh or smoked. Veal, lamb and pork are good too. How to cook them? Easy! In a pressure cooker. You probably have a pressure cooker, now, but may have been neglecting it. If you have one, use it. If not, buy one. You won't regret it. Your meat will retain its savor, it won't shrink a great deal, and if properly prepared, it will be very tender and have a rich gravy.

I prefer the Presto Cooker, made by the National Pressure Cooker Company, in Eau Claire, Wisconsin.

It's easy to use, and seems to me absolutely safe. Mine works like magic I But, of course, any good pressure cooker will give you excellent service.

My method for cooking all of these meats in my cooker is practically the same. Follow the rules for your own cooker. If you haven't a pressure cooker and don't want to buy one, then stew the meat slowly—you'll get good results, even though it will take longer and may not be quite as satisfactory. Sear the meat, the dry fry method. Add garlic and onions, and whatever spices the special recipe calls for. Put it in your cooker and cook according to directions.

Corned beef, heart and tongue do not need to be seared, but they should be soaked before cooking. Meat loaf may be prepared in your cooker or in the oven. Follow your favorite meat recipes! They're almost all suitable for your diet. You've learned, by now, what you'll have to omit. Tomatoes are fine for seasoning. So are herbs and spices. Add no fat, no bread, except high-protein bread, no cream, no rich sauces. That's all!

To make pot roast a real diet dish, cook it hours before you're to serve it—or even the day before. Put it in the refrigerator. When it is cold, skim off all of the fat—it's easy to remove fat then—and reheat. You'll have a nourishing and non-fattening dish. Other meats may be fat-reduced in the same way. So may soups.

Next to meat, eggs, fish and cheese are the chief proteins in a sensible reduction diet. I shall not attempt to tell you how to make an omelet or stuff eggs—you'll undoubtedly know a dozen ways, yourself. Eggs stuffed with diet dressing are excellent. All sorts of omelets, especially mushroom or Spanish omelets, are perfect for diet luncheons.

Here are two fish dishes that I especially like, and that are low in calories—and I don't think you'll find them in your cook books.

23. BAKED FISH IN CHEESE ENVELOPES

Fillets of fish.
Very thin slices of Swiss cheese.
Tomatoes, canned will do.
Accent.
Onions.
Salt substitute.
Garlic.

Fry the onions, cut in large rings, until just soft and light yellow—not brown. Fry with as little fat as possible, or use mineral oil, if allowed, or stew in very little water. Add tomatoes and a bit of garlic, Accent and salt substitute. Stew until some of the moisture has evaporated. Place the pieces of fish in an oiled pan. Bake in medium oven until done— this won't take long. Put a few tablespoons of the tomato and onion on each piece. Cover each portion with a piece of Swiss cheese. Bake until the cheese has melted over each piece. Allow about two pieces for each person. Hearty—and seemingly very hard to make. Looks nice, too. A good main dish when you don't want to serve meat.

24. FISH MOLD

Another company dish—but also fine when you aren't having company, low-calorie and very good. My own invention, too!

2 cans of tuna or salmon. I use the low-calorie tuna.
1 cup cottage cheese.
½ cup water.
2 tablespoons mayonnaise.
1 teaspoon lemon juice.
1 envelope gelatin.
1 teaspoon Worcestershire Sauce.
Salt substitute.
Onion juice, if you like it.

Dissolve the gelatin in cold water. Then heat until it has dissolved. That's all the cooking there is to it! Now add the cottage cheese, and seasonings, and beat until smooth. Then add the fish, flaked, and mixed. Don't mix the fish too smooth—it will taste better if it has substance. If you wish, you can add whole shrimps, too, or garnish with shrimps, though they aren't necessary. You can make this with any kind of cold fish or with crab meat, too, if you like. Experiment with mixtures.

All of the usual fish dishes are good, if they do not contain too many fattening substances—and are not made with too-fat fish.

I've already used cottage cheese in a number of recipes. It is one of the stand-bys of the dieter, rich in all of the life-giving vitamins and minerals that you find in milk. I like pot cheese—which hasn't any cream at all. However, cottage cheese has only a 3 or 4 per cent butterfat content, so if you can't get pot cheese, use cottage cheese. Use the high-calorie cheeses in small quantities, the low-calorie cheeses in large quantities. See your food chart for values. You can't get more for your food money! Most Gouda and Pineapple cheeses are made with partially skimmed milk. There are several other cheeses made with partially skimmed milk, and a large number made with whole milk. Avoid the cheeses made with cream. Farmer's cheese is a good skimmed milk cheese.

25. CHEESE SPREADS

Cottage cheese may be used in a number of spreads, to be eaten with your high-protein breads.

Add a few chopped dates to an 8-ounce cup (½ pound) of cottage cheese and use as a spread. Mix well. Good as your extra snack, with fruit or milk. The Arabs live on milk and dates when they travel, you know. They say it is the perfect food combination.

Add ½ cup pickle relish to a cup of cottage cheese. Good for a change, for canapés, on Melba toast or diet crackers.

Add ¼ cup pimientos to a cup of cottage cheese. This is improved by a little Worcestershire Sauce or mayonnaise.

A very tasty spread can be made by adding, to one cup of cottage cheese, 1 tablespoon of mayonnaise, one small grated onion or onion powder, one cup of chopped watercress—one bunch—and fresh black pepper.

Add ¼ cup diet jelly to cottage cheese, preferably a pink jelly. Beat well. Add a few raisins—not too many! Grated pineapple is good, too.

Add Savita or Boveril—1 tablespoon, plus a little mayonnaise, to 1 cup of cottage cheese. Or a small can of devilled ham.

Add red caviar—or black, if you can afford it—½ cup to 1 cup of cottage cheese. Mix lightly, with a little chopped onion and lemon juice to "point up" the flavor.

All these spreads are best if used a few days after they've been made, so they'll have time to ripen. You'll think up new ones, too. With artichoke toast or gluten bread or crackers, they make nice snacks for those two extra meals, and are good to serve, with drinks, to guests.

I stressed desserts in the beginning, because sweets are so hard to find on a diet. But we all know that, next to our high proteins, vegetables are the most important part of our meals. Do you know how to cook vegetables?

Here is my advice about them: Clean them, using as little water as possible. Rinse well. Do not soak in water, for the vitamins are apt to disappear. Keep in the refrigerator until needed.

Cut the vegetables fine, when possible. Cook in a covered pot, with about ½ inch of water in the bottom of the pot. Cook rapidly. Do not use bicarbonate of soda. Use a little salt—very little. Watch them ! And remove from the stove as soon as they are done. Cabbage can be cooked in less than ten minutes, this way. Turnips will take only a little longer.

Mix them with your butter ration for the day—or with a few drops of mineral oil and one of the flavorings you like. Not too many flavorings, or you'll lose the flavor of the vegetable. Serve large portions of the low-carbohydrate vegetables, and you won't need a great variety at each meal. One, if you have a salad, two if you don't.

26. CELERY STEW

There should be a better name for this. Maybe near-spaghetti. You can use it as a chili con carne base, too. Maybe I'll call it the Think Yourself Thin Stew. It is nourishing, hearty, and low in calories. Tastes good too. What more do you want?

1 can of tomatoes or tomato paste with water.
3 cups of celery, cut crosswise, in ½-inch pieces.
6 medium-sized onions.
1 clove of garlic.
1 carrot, grated.

Fry the onions until a light golden brown—dry fry or use mineral oil. Add garlic, the grated carrot, tomatoes and celery. You may use part Chinese cabbage or regulation cabbage, too. Cook until vegetables are soft.

To vary: Add ½ pound chopped beef.

27. CHILI CON CARNE

Add beef and chili pepper to the celery stew. Then it's imitation chili con carne. If you want a nearer-to-the-real-thing chili, add cooked soya beans. Soak the beans overnight, then cook in a pressure cooker until tender— add to mixture.

Here are some other one-dish meals, with vegetables and meat, that are inexpensive, high in proteins and not too high in calories. All of them may be heated over a second day.

28. HAM AND CABBAGE CASSEROLE

1 cup cooked ground ham.
2 cups shredded cabbage.
2 tablespoons flour.
1 cup skimmed milk.
2 tablespoons grated cheese.

Shred cabbage, and steam in ¼ cup boiling water. Drain. Into heated and greased casserole, place half of cabbage and sprinkle with the flour. Add layer of ham and cover with the remaining cabbage. Pour on heated milk and top with grated cheese. Cover and bake in moderate oven (350°F.) 25 minutes. Remove cover and brown for about 5 minutes. Serves 4 to 6. Steamed rice and buttered asparagus would make this dish an attractive one as well as a well-balanced meal.

29. STUFFED CABBAGE

1 small head cabbage.

½ pound hamburger.

1 onion, chopped.

1 tablespoon fat.

½ cup mashed potato or any cooked cereal.

¼ teaspoon sage or thyme.

Pepper.

Salt substitute.

½ cup milk.

2 slices bacon.

Remove outer leaves of cabbage and arrange over bottom and around sides of a greased casserole. Chop remaining cabbage. Sauté hamburger and onion in fat until onion is tender. Add potato or cereal, seasonings and milk. Turn into cabbage-lined casserole. Cover and bake in a moderate oven (350° F.) fifteen minutes. Remove cover and arrange bacon over top. Continue baking until bacon is crisp, about fifteen minutes.

30. CABBAGE, SAUSAGE AND APPLE CASSEROLE

Shape sausage meat into patties. Preheat a heavy frying pan, place sausage patties in pan, reduce heat to moderate and cook about 12 to13 minutes or until nicely browned on both sides. Pour off grease as it accumulates in pan. Allow about 1½ pounds sausage meat for 6 servings of 2 cakes each. While the sausage is frying, shred 1 medium head cabbage and slice 3 apples. Arrange in layers in a buttered casserole, starting with a layer of cabbage and ending with layer of apples. Place sausage cakes on top. Rinse frying pan in which sausage was fried with 1tablespoon of vinegar and pour over the sausage. Cover and bake in moderate oven (375°F.) about 40 to 45 minutes.

Salads form an important part of your meals while you're on your reduction diet—and all the rest of your life, I hope. If you think Fm going to tell you which vegetables to mix together to make salads, you're mighty mistaken. I've seen whole books—or great sections of books—devoted to telling that very thing. I think you've got sense enough to go to your market and get the vegetables that are in season, or look the freshest, or appeal to you that day, and combine them. That, it seems to me, takes the very least amount of brain power. And you're thinking yourself thin! If you want green peppers, endive and tomato, why should I tell you to have lettuce and cucumbers? Combine any of the raw or cooked vegetables that are on your low-calorie lists. Make up your own salads! You're thinking yourself thin, aren't you? If you run out of ideas, you can look up new combinations in any of the regulation cook books. This isn't the place!

I will give you a couple of good jellied salads, though. There are not so many recipes for those. One is a plain aspic, and can be used for fish, meats and boiled or raw vegetables. The other is a tomato aspic, which can be served alone or with cottage cheese, or you can put vegetables, meat or fish in that, too. Two kinds are all you'll need. You can vary them, too.

31. ASPIC FOR VEGETABLE, MEAT OR FISH SALADS

    1 envelope gelatin.
    ¼, cup cold water.

1⅓cups hot water.
    1   teaspoon whole mixed spices.
    ½ teaspoon salt.
    ⅓ cup vinegar.   Beef cubes, if desired.

Bring water, salt and spices to a boil. Soften gelatin in cold water. Add to hot mixture and stir until dissolved. Add vinegar. Strain and set aside to cool.

32. TOMATO ASPIC

    1 envelope gelatin.
    ¼ cup cold water.
    2 cups tomato juice, canned, or fresh tomatoes.
    2 bay leaves (if desired).
    1 teaspoon salt.
    1 stalk celery, chopped.
    4 teaspoons grated onion.
    Dash cayenne pepper.
    2 tablespoons cider vinegar.
    2 tablespoons lemon juice.

Soften gelatin in cold water. Mix tomato juice or tomatoes with bay leaves, salt, celery, onion, and cayenne pepper. Simmer 10 minutes. Strain. Dissolve gelatin in hot tomato mixture. Add vinegar and lemon juice and turn into large ring mold that has been rinsed in cold water. Chill. When firm, unmold on lettuce and garnish with low-calorie mayonnaise or cooked dressing.

33. DOUBLE-DECKER ASPIC

You can make a most attractive double-decker aspic, by making a cottage cheese mold of:

1 cup cottage cheese.

½ cup water.

1 envelope gelatin.

2 tablespoons of mayonnaise.

Mix water with gelatin. Heat until dissolved. Add cottage cheese and mayonnaise. Serve with vegetables, alone. Or put into a mold and let it get cold, and pour tomato aspic over it, just before the aspic is cold. If you wish the white layer to be as thick as the aspic, double this recipe. A fine company aspic, with or without the addition of vegetables.

Salad dressings are as important as salads. I've seen too many people, who think they are dieting, eat large vegetable salads which are low in calories in themselves, but not when covered with rich French dressings or with mayonnaise, each of which is so high in calories that it turns the dish into one far too fattening for the dieter. Don't fool yourself! Think yourself thin! If you're on a diet, do not use high-calorie salad dressings and ruin your whole diet for the day.

34. BASIC THINK YOURSELF THIN DRESSING

This sounds terrible! I worked it out, myself, and I wouldn't believe it was good if I hadn't made it. I experimented with dozens of dressings. Most of them were

too thin or tasteless. This is fine with almost any vegetable, raw or cooked. Try it.

1 can—two cups—tomato juice or V-Eight.

2 cups cider vinegar.

¼ cup, or a little more, of oil—olive, vegetable or
mineral.

I small onion,

1 clove of garlic.

¼ teaspoon Accent.

1 tablespoon Worcestershire Sauce.

½ teaspoon salad herb blend—I like House of
Herbs brand best.

Paprika.

Salt substitute.

Mix in Waring Blender or electric mixer, until spices
and onion and garlic are well blended. You may add a
tablespoon of sour cream mix No. 2 when you use it, if
you like. Good plain, or with the "cream."

35. THINK YOURSELF THIN THICK DRESSING

This is an extremely low-calorie dressing, a sort of
mayonnaise, that can be used any time that mayonnaise
is needed. It is good as an imitation Hollandaise sauce,
for broccoli, asparagus or any hot vegetable. It is good
with shrimps or meats. It is good with salads. It isn't as
good as a rich mayonnaise or real Hollandaise, but it's
not as fattening, either. In fact, you can use it without
worrying about calories.

1 ½ cups of water.
6 tablespoons cornstarch.
½ cup lemon juice and cider vinegar.
Salt or salt substitute, to taste.
2 Sucaryl or saccharin tablets.
¼ cup oil—vegetable or mineral.
2 teaspoons bottled horseradish.
2½ teaspoons prepared mustard.
1 ½ teaspoons paprika.
1 clove of garlic.
1 teaspoon Worcestershire Sauce.

Cook water and cornstarch until clear and thick—five to six minutes. Take off stove, mix, add rest of ingredients. Beat smooth, using electric mixer, if possible.

Here are two more dressings you may like as a variety.

36. LOW-CALORIE MAYONNAISE

1 egg yolk.
1 teaspoon mustard.
½ teaspoon salt.
1/16 teaspoon paprika.
2 tablespoons cider vinegar.
1 cup mineral oil.
1/16 teaspoon pepper.

Mix mustard, salt, paprika and pepper together, add egg yolk and beat until smooth. Beat in slowly one teaspoonful of vinegar, then beat In oil, drop by drop, until mixture is thick. Then slowly beat in vinegar and oil alternately until both are all used. Keep in jar in refrigerator.

37. LOW-CALORIE COOKED SALAD DRESSING

½ envelope gelatin.
1 egg, well beaten.
4 teaspoons cold water.
¾, cup boiling water.
¼ cup cider vinegar.
1 tablespoon butter.
2 Sucaryl or saccharin tablets.
2 teaspoons mustard.
Salt substitute.
1/16 teaspoon paprika.

Mix together sugar, mustard, salt and paprika. Soften gelatin in cold water. Add boiling water to mustard mixture and stir until smooth. Add softened gelatin and butter, reheat and stir until gelatin is dissolved and butter is melted. Stir slowly hot liquid into beaten egg. Return to stove and stir constantly until mixture begins to thicken. Remove from stove and stir in vinegar. Set aside to cool and thicken.

38. BUTTERMILK SALAD DRESSING

1 pint of buttermilk.
2 Sucaryl or saccharin tablets.
2 tablespoons lemon juice.
2 tablespoons grated onion.
½ chopped garlic clove.

Also parsley, chives, green pepper or celery, chopped fine, if desired—any or all. Shake well, in bottle or jar. Good for fruit or green vegetables.

39. COTTAGE CHEESE DRESSING

This is a fine fruit salad dressing. It can be used with cut fruits, canned or fresh, or with fruit in gelatin.

1 cup cottage cheese.
2 tablespoons oil—any kind.
2 tablespoons lemon juice.
2 tablespoons orange juice or pineapple juice.
Combine ingredients and beat well.

The De Gouy Salad Book, which I've already told you about, has delicious dressings, as well as gourmet aspics, that can easily be adapted to reduction diets, if you use your brains in adapting them—and I'm sure that is easy enough for you to do, now.

40. DIETENE CREAM CUSTARD

Dietene is a reducing supplement, made by the Dietene Company in Minneapolis, Minnesota, for use on a low-calorie reducing diet. It isn't low in calories—100 calories to the ounce—but it is high in protein—about 33%—and contains valuable vitamins as well. It has, however, over 50% carbohydrates. It may be taken in water or milk. I like it as a dessert, as an additional sweet at the end of a meal, where it is needed. Add six tablespoons to 2 cups of water or skimmed milk, in which an envelope of gelatin has been dissolved. Add a pinch of salt or salt substitute, vanilla, a couple of sweet tablets—if you want it very sweet—mix well and chill.

For the last recipes, I can't think of anything more appropriate than ice cream. They are pure sham—for they contain no cream at all. But the first one contains non-fat milk—two kinds—and they are both good for you—as you know well enough, now.

41. NOT-TOO-NEAR ICE CREAM

This is a good frozen dessert. If you like, you may add fruit or "diet preserves" or diet cocoa, when you return it to the freezing tray. Or you may substitute orange juice for part of the milk—in whatever proportion you like—and have a very good orange sherbet. Experiment with this:

½ cup non-fat—dry—skimmed milk.
1 pint skimmed milk.
2 tablespoons flour or cornstarch.
1 egg, separated.
10 tablets Sucaryl or saccharin.
1 teaspoon vanilla.
1 envelope gelatin.
Speck of salt substitute.

Put dry skimmed milk, gelatin and flour into top of double boiler. Add small quantity cold milk, to make paste. Gradually add rest of milk. Heat. Add the well-beaten yoke of egg—gradually, of course. Cook until thickened. Take from fire. Add sweet tablets and vanilla. Freeze in refrigerator tray until mushy. Beat until smooth. Add well beaten white of egg, folding in gently. Freeze for a couple of hours until stiff.

42. COMPANY PINEAPPLE ICE CREAM

Soften 2 teaspoons gelatin in 2 tablespoons cold pineapple juice. Heat to boiling point 1 cup crushed canned pineapple. Stir in 12 sweetening tablets and a bit of salt. Add gelatin and stir until dissolved. Let cool. When mixture thickens, add 2 cups buttermilk, which has been beaten to a foam. Mix thoroughly. Pour into refrigerator trays. When mixture has frozen slightly, remove to chilled bowl and beat until smooth. Beat 1 egg white until stiff and fold into the mixture. Add ½ teaspoon vanilla, return to trays, and freeze. Serves 6.

There ! I think I've given you enough recipes to start you on your way. I think you'll enjoy these. I think you'll enjoy, too, gathering your own diet recipes, as well as your maintenance recipes—not quite so severe, but still low in calories. Part of the fun of thinking yourself thin is knowing what you can and can't eat—and why—and deciding for yourself just what is for you. So, become a real gourmet in your selection of the foods and the recipes for you. And you might send me some glamour recipes, if you find them. Just don't send me a recipe that calls for sliced tomatoes and lettuce, with vinegar poured over them! I know a lot more recipes—but, alas, I haven't room for them here. But I always enjoy good new ones. When I write that cook book . . .

CHAPTER 26

Hold that line!

IT MAY NOT BE the happiest moment in your life—and I hope it isn't; you deserve better—but certainly it is one of the most satisfactory, when you step on the scales in the morning and the indicator stops at exactly the place it should—the perfect weight for you. And when the size of your waistline is exactly what you'd almost been afraid to hope it might be. And you want to yell, "I've made it, Ma!"

You're probably as perfect, physically, as you can get! You have done a good job of improving your appearance, and guarding yourself against disease—of preparing for a long and pleasant future. If you've followed the rules, you look and feel better than you have in years. You should have more energy, more ambition, more sex appeal. You've thought yourself thin!

Now, what are you going to do, once you've reached this much-desired state? If you've learned as much about yourself, and about food and about living, as I hope you have, you'll be able to keep this desirable weight for the rest of your life. If you forget the whole thing and "relapse into error," before too long a time you'll be back where you started, carrying around pounds of superfluous weight, shortening your life, and making yourself prone to a dozen illnesses.

It isn't hard to keep at your right weight, once you have attained it by thinking yourself thin. That I promise you. I traveled through Scandinavia, eating typical Danish, Norwegian and Swedish foods—with only the smallest amount of restraint—and gained only five pounds, shedding them immediately after I got home. I visited Arkansas, my old home, and gained only a few pounds—though I did have to go slow on hot biscuits running over with melted butter, and fried chicken with cream gravy—and lost those pounds quickly, too. But if I'd forgotten the rules, I'm sure I'd have gained—and kept—twenty-five or thirty pounds.

Gypsy Rose Lee, the beautiful authoress, who happens to do a bit of acting and strip teasing as a side-line, tells me that she keeps her practically faultless figure by starting to worry as soon as she gains three pounds.

"I never let fat get more headway than that," she told me. "Then I start to worry. And to diet. I cut out all fattening foods at once—before fat has a chance to accumulate. In a few days, I'm at my normal weight again. Once you let fat get the upper hand, you have a far more difficult time."

The other day, a man said to me, "It's easy enough for me to lose. I don't need any fancy diets! All I do is give up starches and sweets."

"That's very sensible," I said, "for then, unconsciously, you're turning to proteins."

"Of course I am! No fancy diets for me!"

"That's fine!" I said. "Then you haven't any weight problems."

"Oh, yes I have," he told me. "As soon as I stop dieting, I begin to gain. Just a little—or none at all the first few weeks, while I'm careful. But then, as I grow hungry or careless, I gain more and more—until I've gained back all I've lost."

"Then what?" I asked.

"Oh, then I start in dieting all over again."

I tried to tell him that that seemed sort of silly. He didn't get the idea. I hope you do. Why torture your system by dieting—and then gaining and then dieting again?

The ideal way to diet, as I hope you've learned, is to understand yourself. And to eat the foods that are good for you. They can be, as you've found out, well-seasoned, well-balanced and of a good variety. Once you've reached your ideal weight, add just enough good food to your diet to maintain that weight. You're normal now—and should stay that way.

The main thing about losing weight, and then maintaining your ideal weight, is an understanding of yourself. Know why you were fat. And realize how you conquered that fat. And how you can keep the fat at bay.

Obese people are sick people. And food makes fat. It's as simple as that. Once you are slender—and have become slender through sensible treatment of your body—

then you have conquered your illness—you are well, again. But you are still obesity prone! Probably you are still far more apt to gain fat than the person who is not obesity prone. Whether you have a tendency to be fat because of heredity or because you love food, the original basic reason may still be existent. You have conquered your desire—for the time being. Perhaps you have conquered it forever. I hope so. But you must be on^ the lookout all the time. Forever? Certainly! But it isn't as difficult as you'd think, once you put your mind to it. Practically every star on the stage or screen is "careful," when it comes to diet.

If you have heart trouble, you know there are certain things you can or cannot do. High blood pressure requires certain treatment. Your obesity must be treated with the same deference. Fat stay away from my door!

You'll have certain temptations. Temptations make you stronger—if you resist them. It's fun resisting temptation, once you get used to it.

There's that food orgy! Once you've reduced down to size, there's a great desire to throw off all restrictions and sit down to a Lucullan feast. Don't do it! For a lot of reasons. You may not actually gain weight on one Diamond Jim Brady feast. But it will break down the resistance you've built up. You won't be a bit better off for it. I can guarantee that! If you want a feast, try a steak with a big baked potato, eating not too much of the fat And don't drink water with the meal! Have a salad or a green vegetable with it. And for dessert, have fruit, cheese and crackers, or a small portion of ice cream. For a first course, you may have shrimps, fish, crab meat, oysters or a mixed hors d'oeuvres. Isn't that feast enough? You may substitute any baked meat, poultry or fish for the steak, if you—or your purse—prefer. And you won't gain weight or destroy your good habits of eating, either.

Those cocktail parties! They are a great temptation for anyone not on a strict diet. While you're dieting, it is easy enough to stay away from cocktail temptations. Once you're off that, it is so easy to reach out for those forbidden goodies you've been denying yourself—sausages in pastry covering, little hot miniature cheese pies, nuts, potato chips, caviar canapés—all good, and all top-heavy with calories. If you like, eat five or six canapés and have two cocktails—and go without your dinner! Those canapés actually may have about 100 calories each, the bread 25 calories, the butter another 25 calories, and the topping—of paté or rich creamed food—can easily add another 50 calories each—six of these, and two cocktails and you have eaten what could have been a satisfying meal. Sometimes—if you insist—a cocktail party can be indulged in—if you'll skip dinner. If you still want to eat dinner, then keep down to one or two canapes and one, or at most two, cocktails. You'll be better off without the many "sips and nibbles." But if you insist on them . . .

"My chief trouble is when I dine at a friend's home, once I'm no longer on a strict diet," a friend told me, recently. "My hostess gets furious, if I don't eat! And the food looks so good."

But you can eat—and liberally, too, if you're the least bit careful! Once you are not trying to lose weight, you may have practically anything except the most concentrated and fattening foods. Eat a medium-sized helping of potatoes—but go slow on the rich gravy, which you probably won't crave anymore, anyway. Try not to drink water with your dinner—which will keep you from eating too much, too. Go slow on hot breads, rich salad dressings and rich desserts! Take as large a portion of meat as seems polite, and enjoy that and the vegetables. If you don't make a point of it, your hostess won't notice that you aren't eating everything. The only foods you must refuse, or take in small portions, are the usual servings of soup, spaghetti, macaroni, pancakes, sauces and desserts.

You'll have no problem when you eat in restaurants. Look at your pages for reduction while eating out—and add a bit to those. You'll be generously fed. When you eat at home, your problem is solved, too. Larger portions, or one of the foods you've been denying yourself, added to your reduction diet, and you're all set for generous meals.

The diet you must have now is a general, well-balanced diet—suitable for everyone who wants to stay well, and look well. You don't have to "cater to yourself." You can practically forget that you are dieting at all. In fact, you'll be eating what are considered by experts the necessary foods for good nutrition. Your diet should include the seven basic groups of foods, in the following proportions :

1. Leafy green and yellow vegetables—one or more servings each day.

2. Citrus fruits or other foods high in Vitamin C—one or more servings—see your Vitamin and Calorie lists.

3. Potatoes and other vegetables and fruits—two servings per day.

4. Milk—two cups per day—one pint of whole milk, skimmed milk or buttermilk.

5. Meat, poultry or fish—one generous serving. Eggs —4 or more per week. When eggs are not used, add peas, nuts, peanut butter or cheese, especially cottage cheese, to your menus.

6. Whole wheat, gluten or enriched bread, one or two slices.

7. Butter, fortified margarine or olive oil daily.

These are the needed foods. In addition, you may probably have light desserts, some jam or jelly, olives, pickles and spices, as well as a moderate amount of sauces and salad dressings.

How will you know how much to eat? That is something that only you, yourself, can find. The way to find the amount that you need is to add the above foods to your diet in small amounts, until you have found your maintenance diet. It may vary from 1,500 to 3,000 calories a day.

How to find your maintenance diet is the simplest

thing in the world. Please continue to "weigh in" every morning. And to write down what you eat every night. Those two habits are as necessary, now, to keep your correct weight, as they were when you were thinking yourself thin. By watching your weight and your food intake, you can tell, immediately, if you are eating too much—or choosing the wrong foods for you. As soon as you find that you've gained, even if it is only a fraction of a pound, cut out the unnecessary food, the added goodies. Lose that extra weight at once!

By this time you should know yourself. And you should know foods. It is impossible for anyone to tell exactly how much you may eat on a maintenance diet. But it is possible to tell you the foods that are good for you. Stick to those "basic seven" and you'll be eating for health—and getting good food, too.

I can't tell you what to eat at each meal—and I'm sure you wouldn't want me to. Use your own judgment, tastes and dietary habits in choosing your food, as long as you keep to the basic rules. Here is a day's diet. It is not given for you to follow blindly, but just to show you what you may have that is good—and good for you. These are examples only. Make up your own menus!

Your breakfast, if well-balanced, should consist of fruit, a cereal or eggs, bread and butter, and coffee and milk, or not-too-rich cream. You might have:

Grapefruit
Whole grain cereal, with milk or thin cream

or

Soft boiled eggs,
Whole wheat or gluten toast and butter
Coffee

For luncheon, you might have meat or a substitute, a vegetable, salad with dressing, a light dessert, bread and butter. If you have a starchy vegetable at luncheon, omit it at dinner. The same goes for a fairly heavy dessert. Here is a typical luncheon:

Cold sliced ham with potato salad

or

Hot meat with green vegetables

or

Salad with cottage cheese

or

A substantial sandwich Celery and
carrots Fruit—pear or banana or
apple or gelatin

For dinner, you'll probably want a first course, meat, potatoes or rice, vegetables, salad, and dessert. Here is a good menu, which you may vary in a hundred ways:

Shrimps or crab meat
Roast beef Mashed
potatoes String beans

Sliced tomatoes and lettuce
Vanilla ice cream
Whole wheat bread and butter

These menus may be too generous for you. They are for me! I can't eat three such hearty meals without gaining weight. But I like a "nibble" at four or five o'clock in the afternoon—and a bit of food before I go to bed at night. I prefer an apple and "special" cheese at night, and a small sandwich or cookie and tea at four. You must find your own menus, based on your own tastes and your own needs.

All of the things you've learned about nutrition and vitamins are as important to you now as they were when you were trying to lose weight. In a way, a knowledge of food content is more important once you have reached your perfect weight than while you are losing weight, for continual health and good looks.

You see, you can lose on practically any reduction diet. A diet of eggs for breakfast, meat for luncheon and fruit for dinner—a diet recommended as "new"—will reduce you. But so will any of the diets you've heard about, from starvation diets to diets that are good for you —and including those too low in valuable nutriments. They will reduce you—but they may not help you get a proper food balance, or put you in permanent good condition. More than that, they leave you very hungry and unsatisfied.

However, if you lose on the Think Yourself Thin diet, you've had the foods you need for health and attraction. You've dieted in a way that could not hurt you, but undoubtedly has helped you find health and a sense of well-being. So, once you've reached your right weight, you won't rush into a restaurant, mutter "Thank goodness that's over!"—and begin to gorge on forbidden foods. You'll be well fed on good proteins and vitamins. While you'll be glad to add some calories to your daily intake, and will enjoy the "extras," you shouldn't feel starved or mistreated—and you shouldn't go overboard by unwise stuffing.

After you've reached your right weight, you'll want to keep on with your exercise and massage. That ten minutes a day of exercise should have become a habit, by now. Surely ten or fifteen minutes of your time isn't too much to spend on keeping supple and fit. Your body, now, should be firm and not flabby, for you should have lost gradually, and exercised enough to make your muscles stronger—taken up the "slack" that the weight loss might have caused without exercise. You'll want to continue your facial exercises for appearance' sake, too.

Once you've lost weight, I think you'll enjoy long walks. You're no longer carrying around pounds of superfluous weight, and your step should be springy and young. Your walks should not be a substitute for that ten minutes of stretching and bending, but a good supplement. You'll get new ideas while walking, too. And any ideas that will take you out of yourself are good.

Keep up your daily hot and cold bath. It is the best possible way to stimulate your body—to make you look and feel well. If possible, take a hot shower after your stretching and bending exercises. Then take as cold a shower as you can stand. Rub your skin until it glows, with a rough bath towel. Don't neglect your face and neck! The hot and cold water, plus rubbing with a rough towel, will help your facial as well as body circulation.

You have learned the relation between mental and physical well-being. Only by learning about yourself and understanding yourself can you grow slender in the right way—and stay slender the right way. You've learned, I hope, how to think yourself thin. Now, by thinking yourself thin, you can retain that weight—and retain it for a long and, I hope, contented and successful life.

How are your teeth? They have a lot more to do with your looking well and young—and being well and young—than you may believe. First, for appearance' sake. If your teeth are yellow or have fillings in front or are broken, they undoubtedly detract from your appearance, make you look older than you are. Today, with the many plastic jacket crowns that are being manufactured, you owe it to yourself, to have your teeth crowned if they do not look well. No longer will they have to look like a row of white porcelain. They'll look the way your teeth would look if you were looking your best.

Hollywood dentists have a way of equipping all stars, young and old, with new sets of jacket crowns, if their own teeth fall short of perfection. And they use "buttons" or plumpers, if age gives them fallen cheeks. You may not need to look like a movie star. But you do need to look the best—and most natural—for you.

But teeth are more important than that. Teeth actually can make you ill, or help keep you well. You know, of course, that absessed or diseased teeth cause germs to go through your system—drag you down. But you may not have absesses at all. Perhaps you've lost teeth and can't chew well. That will interfere with your looks, with your digestion, and with your ability to follow a diet. I went to Dr. Irving Goldman, dental surgeon, lecturer and contributor to medical and dental journals, and asked him to stress the importance of good teeth. Dr. Goldman believes that if teeth are worn short of full form, they should be fixed, the "bite raised," for looks and health. Dr. Goldman told me:

"Good tone of the facial tissues only results when the underlying muscles achieve their fullest function. This is possible when we have healthy teeth in healthy gums, in a good mechanical arrangement for effective mastication."

So—see your dentist. He can be as important as your doctor in bringing you up to par—and in allowing you to get the most out of life while you're thinking yourself thin and forgetting all about age.

What about plastic surgery? Here is something you must decide for yourself. I've seen remarkable results. Certainly, if your nose is out of joint, literally, a plastic operation may rid you of an ugly proboscis and a bad inferiority complex. Oversized breasts are often operated on. This means about two weeks in a hospital, and is major surgery. Face lifts take long strips of skin from around the hairline—do away with superfluous skin. They do not touch the muscles. If done by a good surgeon they can be most effective—for a while. Of course, face lifts do not last forever, but some people, especially professionals who must have smooth faces, find the operation well worth while. All plastic operations have lost the dread secrecy that used to surround them. Today, if you need them and want them badly enough, why, you may have them. Never have a plastic operation without the recommendation and full cooperation of your own physician, whom you know and trust. A bad plastic surgeon could ruin your appearance forever. Exercise and diet, and the right treatment of your face and body, may do just the things for you that you hoped to accomplish by plastic surgery. Follow my rules, first, and see what happens. You may not need anything more drastic.

By thinking, you have become the person you wanted to be. It's an easy matter to stay that way. Your chief difficulties are over. Now you can enjoy the fruits of your labor. You'll receive the compliments of your friends. You'll have new attraction and charm. You'll have a new sense of accomplishment and satisfaction.

Forget about food, except when you are planning menus, studying your own charts, cooking or eating. The rest of the time, turn your mind to the hundreds of interesting things around you.

Feed yourself, and your family and your guests, the best foods you can get—and you know now what these foods are. Eat in moderation. And give out as much happiness with your meals—and other times, too—as you can.

Keep the corners of your mouth up. Hold your shoulders back, your stomach in, your head high. Make new friends—and don't be afraid to give to them, in happiness and inspiration. Keep your thoughts on the things that are important for you today and tomorrow.

And remember that your body is you—as much as your brain is you. It is so easy to feel that we are just a brain— a thinking machine—-and that our body does not belong to us at all. If we realize that our bodies are as much a part of us as our brains, it will be easier to fit into our world, to be better citizens—even to eat more sensibly. Every bite you eat becomes you. Every thought you think is tied up with your whole being. Wherever you go you are judged, not by your mind, but by yourself as a whole—by your physical being. So what you eat actually represents you—not that you are a gourmet or a glutton, but the physical you, as you impress people who meet you, for the first or the thousandth time. Live and eat and think so that you can give to the world the impression of you as you would like to be.

Try to make the part of the world that touches you a little better than it would be without you. Nothing to do with being slender? Try it I Try forgetting about fears, about insecurity. Think yourself into being the person you've always wanted to be. Think positive and good thoughts. I think I can promise you that, if you'll follow these rules, you'll be thinking yourself into happiness as well as into physical improvement.

Once you have shed your fat, which formed a sort of disguise and kept you from presenting the real you to the world—and to yourself—you'll find a new enjoyment in living, new incentives for success. You'll have gained new self-confidence with your new appearance, and shed your inferiority complex with those unnecessary pounds. You've proved to yourself—and to the world—that you have the necessary strength of character to attain what you set out for—a sound, firm and well-proportioned body. You'll be pleasing to look at—and therefore more pleasing to be with. You'll like yourself better as other people like you better. And you've gained health—and the opportunity for continued health—as you've attained your correct weight.

By losing weight, you've gained in every other way. You've joined a notable company of people who have found new happiness in new figures. And success and contentment they never dreamed possible while they were overweight. Here are my best wishes while, and after, you think yourself thin.

new self-confidence with your new appearance, and shed your inferiority complex with those unnecessary pounds. You've proved to yourself—and to the world—that you have the necessary strength of character to attain what you set out for—a sound, firm and well-proportioned body. You'll be pleasing to look at—and therefore more pleasing to be with. You'll like yourself better as other people like you better. And you've gained health—and the opportunity for continued health—as you've attained your correct weight.

By losing weight, you've gained in every other way. You've joined a notable company of people who have found new happiness in new figures. And success and contentment they never dreamed possible while they were overweight. Here are my best wishes while, and after, you think yourself thin.

Also available from www.sunvillagepublications.com

Eat All You Want And Watch
Your Fat Melt Quickly Away
With Fredrick Kerr's...

HIGH
PROTEIN
DIET

By Fredrick Kerr
With An Introduction By
Leonid Kotkin M.D.